Controlling and Preventing Errors in Nursing Care of Pediatric Patients

Kim Maryniak

Controlling and Preventing Errors in Nursing Care of Pediatric Patients

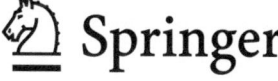

Kim Maryniak
Independent Consultant
Casa Grande, AZ, USA

Editorial Contact: Marie-Elia Come-Garry

ISBN 978-3-031-88184-8   ISBN 978-3-031-88185-5 (eBook)
https://doi.org/10.1007/978-3-031-88185-5

© The Editor(s) (if applicable) and The Author(s), under exclusive license to Springer Nature Switzerland AG 2025

This work is subject to copyright. All rights are solely and exclusively licensed by the Publisher, whether the whole or part of the material is concerned, specifically the rights of translation, reprinting, reuse of illustrations, recitation, broadcasting, reproduction on microfilms or in any other physical way, and transmission or information storage and retrieval, electronic adaptation, computer software, or by similar or dissimilar methodology now known or hereafter developed.

The use of general descriptive names, registered names, trademarks, service marks, etc. in this publication does not imply, even in the absence of a specific statement, that such names are exempt from the relevant protective laws and regulations and therefore free for general use.

The publisher, the authors and the editors are safe to assume that the advice and information in this book are believed to be true and accurate at the date of publication. Neither the publisher nor the authors or the editors give a warranty, expressed or implied, with respect to the material contained herein or for any errors or omissions that may have been made. The publisher remains neutral with regard to jurisdictional claims in published maps and institutional affiliations.

This Springer imprint is published by the registered company Springer Nature Switzerland AG
The registered company address is: Gewerbestrasse 11, 6330 Cham, Switzerland

If disposing of this product, please recycle the paper.

Special thanks to our peer reviewers:

Natalie McPherson, BSN, RNC-NIC

Angie Bannochie, MSN, BSN, RNC-NIC

Introduction

Pediatric patients are generally those from birth through age 18, although there are also considerations through age 21, and with patients who have developmental delays (Strouse et al., 2022). Pediatrics are considered a vulnerable population, requiring specific knowledge and care. An error that occurs with a child has the potential to range from minor to severe, has life-long irreversible consequences, or can even be fatal. Nurses have the greatest role in direct patient care, and as members of the most trusted profession have a responsibility to avoid errors and protect these defenseless patients. During this time of global staffing shortages, pediatric patients are sicker and more acute, and additionally, there are more task-oriented duties assigned to nurses. These factors can create imbalances and create an overwhelming workload. The aim of *Controlling and Preventing Errors in Nursing Care of Pediatric Patients* is to inform nurses about the most common and the more serious errors made in caring for pediatric patients. This book covers topics about the uniqueness of pediatric patients and common conditions that are seen with patients in pediatric settings.

This book explores a variety of pediatric conditions related to developmental levels, including infectious diseases, jaundice, cardiac anomalies, respiratory illnesses, fluid and electrolyte imbalances, pediatric cancers, diabetes, sepsis, behavioral disorders, and trauma. Causes, signs, and management of these conditions are discussed. The types of errors, consequences, detection, and monitoring for nursing errors are included. There are multiple types of errors that can occur during the care of pediatric patients related to handling, assessment, and treatment. Medication errors can also occur which can have detrimental consequences. Multiple negative outcomes can arise from nursing errors, affecting the patient, family, and even the healthcare professionals involved. Negative effects at an organization-wide level may also occur as a result of errors.

There are a variety of strategies that can be implemented to detect and monitor for nursing errors. Process improvement and quality assurance through use of effective tools can assist with detection and monitoring of errors. System tactics and effective communication are also vital to make improvements. A workplace culture that is supportive with effective leadership can also assist in reduction of errors.

Application of just culture is discussed, and how that framework can be used to determine cause of errors, as well as the potential need for system and process improvements. Predisposing and contributing factors for nursing errors will be reviewed, which can include personal factors, such as health or knowledge, processes, and environmental factors. Often a combination of factors can exist, which can create a higher risk for errors.

The book describes how errors can be avoided with necessary precautions, and managed appropriately based on current evidence-based practice. There are many practices that have been identified in studies to help prevent nursing errors, such as the use of bundles to prevent hospital-acquired conditions. System and personal considerations can also prevent nursing errors.

Case studies and examples are provided, demonstrating effective practices for reducing patient errors with pediatric patients. Recommendations for further study are also provided.

Reference

Strouse, P.J., Trout, A.T., & Offiah, A.C. (2022). Editors' notebook: What is 'pediatric'? *Pediatric Radiology, 52*(12), 2241–2242.

Contents

1 Overview of Common Conditions in Pediatric Patients 1
   Infants 1
      Respiratory Syncytial Virus (RSV) and Bronchiolitis............................ 2
      Acute Respiratory Failure..................... 3
      Infections and Sepsis......................... 3
      Hyperbilirubinemia.......................... 5
   Gastroenteritis................................ 7
   Cardiac Disorders 7
   Toddlers...................................... 20
      Pneumonia.................................. 21
      Bronchitis 22
      Asthma 22
      Acute Respiratory Failure..................... 23
      Fluid and Electrolyte Imbalance................ 23
      Infections.................................. 25
      Seizures and Epilepsy........................ 27
      Pediatric Cancer 27
   Pre-school Aged Children....................... 29
      Infections.................................. 30
      Respiratory Illnesses......................... 30
      Pediatric Cancer 33
      Seizures and Epilepsy........................ 34
      Diabetes................................... 34

	School-Aged Children	36
	Diabetes	37
	Pediatric Cancer	37
	Respiratory Illness	38
	Seizures and Epilepsy	38
	Appendicitis	38
	Infections and Sepsis	38
	Adolescents	39
	Behavioral Disorders	40
	Anxiety, Depression, and Suicidal Ideation	41
	Trauma	42
	Seizures and Epilepsy	43
	Cancer	43
	Appendicitis	43
	Diabetes	44
	References	44
2	**Predisposing and Contributing Factors for Nursing Errors**	49
	References	53
3	**Types of Errors**	55
	Errors Associated with Hospital-Acquired Conditions	56
	Errors Associated with Developmental Stages	58
	Errors Associated with Medical Devices and Equipment	59
	Errors Associated with Identification	60
	Errors Related to Procedures	60
	Errors Affecting Skin Integrity	61
	Medication Errors	61
	Errors Related to Missed Nursing Care	62
	References	62
4	**Consequences of Nursing Errors**	65
	Levels of Harm	65
	Avoidable Harm	67
	Long-Term Harmful Effects	68

	Central Line–Associated Blood Stream Infections. . . .	68
	Catheter-Associated Urinary Tract Infections.	69
	Ventilator-Associated Pneumonia.	69
	Disruption of Skin Integrity	70
	Harm from Medication Errors	70
	The Impact of Falls.	71
	Widespread Effects of Patient Harm.	71
	References.	72
5	**Monitoring for and Detecting Nursing Errors**.	75
	References.	84
6	**Best Practices to Prevent Nursing Errors**.	85
	Scope of Practice.	85
	Bedside Report	86
	Interdisciplinary Rounding	87
	Standardized Communication.	88
	Strategies Specific to Infection Prevention	89
	Approaches for Preventing CLABSIs.	92
	Best Practices for Avoiding CAUTIs	92
	Preventing Ventilator-Associated Pneumonia.	93
	Strategies for Preventing Pressure Injuries	94
	Fall Prevention Strategies	95
	Strategies for Preventing Medication Errors.	96
	Using a Daily Management System	103
	References.	105
7	**Case Studies**.	107
	Case Study #1	107
	Case Study #2	110
	Summary.	111
	Reference	111
8	**Recommendations for Further Study**	113
	References.	114

Summary 115

Overview of Common Conditions in Pediatric Patients

Infants

A baby from birth to about one year of age is referred to as an infant, and physical health and developmental milestones are key areas of focus at this stage. Initially, infants are only able to communicate by crying and non-verbal cues to show pain, discomfort, or hunger. Mimicking sounds and speaking a few words occur during the first year, and they can also comply with simple commands and handle objects near the end of this stage. Infants are completely dependent on the care of others (Maryniak, 2019).

According to Erikson, trust versus mistrust is the stage of development for an infant. The primary task is to develop trust in their caregivers and the environment (Balasundaram & Avulakunta, 2023). Failure to thrive may occur in an infant who fails to develop trust.

Infants need to have their needs met in a timely manner and human touch and contact is important. Nurses can promote bonding between caregivers and infants by having caregivers assist with infant care. Fear of separation can be decreased with participation of caregivers and by remaining in the infant's view. To minimize stranger anxiety, another strategy is by practicing primary nursing to limit how many staff members participate in the care of each infant.

© The Author(s), under exclusive license to Springer Nature Switzerland AG 2025
K. Maryniak, *Controlling and Preventing Errors in Nursing Care of Pediatric Patients*, https://doi.org/10.1007/978-3-031-88185-5_1

Safety is essential for infants because they are dependent. Safe, age-appropriate toys that stimulate motor skills and cognitive development can be used with supervision. Unsafe items such as medications and small objects should always be kept out of the reach of infants. Safety precautions are also required in the environment, such as preventing access to cords or equipment.

Respiratory Syncytial Virus (RSV) and Bronchiolitis

The human respiratory syncytial virus (RSV) is one of the most common causes of bronchiolitis in children globally (Jain et al., 2023; Justice et al., 2023). This virus is highly contagious via respiratory droplets and does not create immunity after exposure, which increases the likelihood of reinfection. RSV can cause upper and lower respiratory illness, the most common of which is bronchiolitis. Bronchiolitis is an infection in the lower airways, which can also create small airway obstructions. The infection is generally self-limited but can progress to respiratory failure, particularly in infants. Risk factors for more severe illness include prematurity, infants younger than three months of age, immunodeficiency, neuromuscular or cardiovascular disease, and chronic lung disease (or bronchopulmonary dysplasia). Vaccinations are available to protect against RSV and are especially recommended for those who have risk factors (Jain et al., 2023; Justice et al., 2023).

Symptoms of RSV include rhinorrhea, cough, sneezing, nasal congestion, myalgia, and fever. Progression to lower airway infection such as bronchiolitis includes symptoms of wheezing, crackles, rhonchi, tachypnea, retractions, grunting, cyanosis. Irritability and poor feeding are also associated (Jain et al., 2023; Justice et al., 2023).

Management of RSV and bronchiolitis are based on symptoms and include intensive fluid and hydration. Nasal saline, cool mist humidifiers, and antipyretics are also used. Humidified oxygen may also be needed. Severe respiratory distress may warrant intensive care monitoring and respiratory management (Jain et al., 2023; Justice et al., 2023).

Acute Respiratory Failure

Infections, diseases, or disorders can cause respiratory distress or failure, particularly in infants. Acute respiratory failure (ARF) is a sudden failure of the respiratory system to maintain adequate gas exchange, requiring immediate intervention. ARF requires intensive care and is one of the most common causes of cardiopulmonary arrest in pediatrics (Panetti et al., 2024). Common causes of respiratory failure for infants include pneumonia, bronchiolitis, neuromuscular diseases, and chronic lung disease. Infants are also more susceptible to developing ARF as a result of respiratory system anatomy and physiology (Panetti et al., 2024).

Symptoms of respiratory failure include respiratory distress, such as retractions, use of accessory muscles, tachypnea, labored breathing, irregular respirations, changes in alertness or consciousness, and abnormal levels of blood oxygen and carbon dioxide concentrations. Pulse oximetry, capnography, and blood gas analyses are important to identify ARF and the severity of the condition. Chest x-rays are also used to diagnose ARF (Panetti et al., 2024; Springer, 2022).

Management of respiratory failure include oxygenation and ventilatory support. Airway management, patient positioning, and mechanical ventilation are typical strategies for ARF. Extracorporeal membrane oxygenation (ECMO) may also be required in severe cases. Monitoring pulse oximetry, capnography, and blood gases are also needed (Springer, 2022). Medications such as steroids, antiviral, or antibiotics may be used to treat underlying conditions. Surfactant may also be beneficial (Panetti et al., 2024; Springer, 2022).

Infections and Sepsis

Infections are commonly seen in infants and particularly neonates within the first 30 days of life, due to their susceptibility from immature protective mechanisms, breaches in the line of defense from invasive procedures, and contact with potential contaminants from the vagina and the environment. There are also multiple risk factors for developing infections in the neonate, including maternal, neonatal, and other factors. Maternal risk factors are premature labor, fever, urinary tract infection, chorioamnionitis, group B strep positive or unknown status, premature or prolonged rupture of membranes, prolonged or difficult labor, poor prenatal care, lower socioeconomic status, inadequate nutrition, multiple pregnancy, and substance abuse. Neonatal risk factors are congenital anomalies, fetal distress, asphyxia, meconium aspiration, prematurity, low birthweight, and inborn errors of metabolism. Other risk factors for infection are resuscitation, invasive procedures, length of hospitalization, use of anti-infective medications, delayed enteral feedings, and total parenteral nutrition (Maryniak, 2023; Singh et al., 2022).

The cause of sepsis is the spread of invading organisms and any byproducts through the bloodstream and tissues. These organisms can be bacterial, viral, fungal, or parasitic organisms. Early-onset sepsis occurs within the first 72 hours of life from maternal transmission during pregnancy or delivery, or immediately following delivery, with group-B strep being the most common cause. Late-onset sepsis happens after 72 hours of age. Congenital viral infections are classified using the TORCH acronym: T—toxoplasmosis, O—other (syphilis, varicella, parvovirus, human immunodeficiency virus, enterovirus), R—rubella, C—cytomegalovirus (CMV), and H—herpes simplex. Other common infections that can lead to sepsis in the infant include urinary tract and kidney infections, central line infections, gastrointestinal tube infections, and perforations, to name a few (Maryniak, 2023; Freedman et al., 2024).

General signs of infections and sepsis are seen in early and late stages. Early signs include apnea, tachypnea, increased oxygen requirements, tachycardia, widened pulse pressure, flushing, full pulses, lethargy, hypotonia, temperature instability, behavioral changes, feeding intolerance, metabolic acidosis, glucose instability, either increased or decreased total white blood cells, an increased immature to total (I:T) white blood cell ratio, and thrombocytopenia. Signs in late stage are decreased systolic pressure, narrowing of pulse pressure, renal failure, splenomegaly, hepatomegaly, seizures, multiple organ dysfunction syndrome, lactic acidosis, higher blood urea nitrogen (BUN) and creatinine, and hyperbilirubinemia.

Management of infections and sepsis depends on the causative organism, stage of the infection, and comorbidities. Anti-infectives are given based on the invading organism. Other strategies are maintenance of a neutral thermal environment, isolation, fluid and electrolyte balance, adequate oxygenation and ventilation, supporting perfusion, removal of central lines, exchange transfusion, and administration of intravenous immunoglobulin (IVIG) (Maryniak, 2023; Miranda & Nadel, 2023).

Hyperbilirubinemia

Bilirubin is the natural byproduct of dying red blood cells, which is transported to the liver by binding with albumin. Bound bilirubin is considered non-toxic. The liver conjugates bilirubin to break it down and eliminate it through the stool. If albumin binding sites are saturated, unconjugated bilirubin becomes free bilirubin, circulating in the blood, which can cross the blood-brain barrier, and become toxic. As the bilirubin production exceeds the liver's capacity to clear it, jaundice develops. Hyperbilirubinemia is seen with prematurity, small for gestational age (SGA), microcephaly, extravascular blood (such as hematoma and bruising), ABO incompatibility, pallor, petechiae, hepatosplenomegaly, chorioretinitis, and hypothyroidism (Kemper et al., 2022; Maryniak, 2023).

Hyperbilirubinemia presents with several signs, and the most commonly seen is jaundice, which progresses in a cephalocaudal direction. Kernicterus, or bilirubin encephalopathy, is a syndrome of severe brain damage caused by unconjugated bilirubin deposited in the brain cells. Unconjugated bilirubin is highly toxic to neurons because of fat-soluble affinity for fatty tissues. There is no treatment for kernicterus. Signs of kernicterus are lethargy, hypotonia, poor suck and ability to feed, high-pitched cry, irritability, moderate stupor, hypertonia, inability to handle stimulation, arching of neck or back, fever, deep stupor to coma, and dystonia (Kemper et al., 2022; Maryniak, 2023).

There are several tests to evaluate hyperbilirubinemia, including total serum bilirubin and direct (conjugated bilirubin). Transcutaneous bilirubin checks are reliable for estimates of serum bilirubin but may limit accuracy depending on skin pigmentation, postnatal age, gestational age and weight of infant. Blood type and direct Coomb's test are testing for isoimmune hemolytic disease and ABO incompatibility. Other tests are blood type, hematocrit, Rh and antibody of screen (Kemper et al., 2022; Maryniak, 2023).

Management of hyperbilirubinemia is essential for prevention of bilirubin encephalopathy, and is dependent on the etiology, age, and bilirubin levels. Strategies may include early initiation of feeding, frequent breastfeeding, adequate fluid balance, phototherapy, intravenous immunoglobulin (IVIG) administration, and exchange transfusion, if indicated.

Phototherapy is the use of ultraviolet lights on exposed skin, which promotes bilirubin excretion by photoisomerization and alters the structure of bilirubin to a water-soluble form for easier excretion. For effective phototherapy, the neonate's skin must be as exposed as possible to light source, using eye shields to protect the eyes from light. During phototherapy, eye checks should be done with feedings to assess for discharge, pressure, and irritation. There are several potential side effects from phototherapy, such as loose stools, transient skin rashes, hyperthermia, higher metabolic rate, insensible water loss, dehydration, electrolyte imbalances, lethargy, and eye damage (Kemper et al., 2022; Maryniak, 2023).

IVIG administration is used when neonates have hemolytic disease as a result of ABO incompatibility. Neonates who have hyperbilirubinemia with hemolytic disease can have a decreased need for an exchange transfusion by infusion of IVIG. Management of these neonates include use of phototherapy in addition to IVIG administration. Less than four doses of IVIG is recommended, which demonstrate good results (Zohreh Jalali et al., 2024).

Exchange transfusions may be indicated for significant hemolytic disease, based on condition and age of the neonate, or if phototherapy fails. An exchange transfusion is done in small aliquots over several hours, removing partially hemolyzed red blood cells and replacing them with donor red blood cells. As the bilirubin is removed, the unbound bilirubin quickly attaches to the unbound donor albumin. Exchange transfusions may cause complications, such as electrolyte and acid-base imbalances, temperature imbalance, necrotizing enterocolitis, vasospasms, thrombi or emboli, infarctions, arrhythmias, volume overload, blood pressure variances, infection, and graft-versus-host disease (Maryniak, 2023; Kemper et al., 2022).

Gastroenteritis

Gastroenteritis generally occurs from various pathogens, including viral, bacterial, and parasitic strains. There are also forms of gastroenteritis that are from non-infectious causes. The most common reason for hospitalizations of infants with gastroenteritis is the dehydration associated with diarrhea and vomiting. In gastroenteritis, the intestinal villi are damaged and release of toxins from infectious sources create diarrhea. Viral infection, particularly the rotavirus, is the most frequent cause of gastroenteritis, responsible for more than 35% worldwide of deaths resulting from diarrhea (Prescilla, 2023).

Management of gastroenteritis primarily focuses on rehydration of the infant. When infants are breastfeeding, it is important to continue feeding. Oral rehydration solutions, including use through nasogastric tubes, if needed, are an important treatment of dehydration. Intravenous (IV) therapy may also be warranted in the hospitalized infant. Use of antidiarrheal medication is contraindicated in gastroenteritis. Antibiotics are only indicated when the cause of gastroenteritis is bacterial. Antiemetics are warranted when the infant is vomiting (Prescilla, 2023).

Cardiac Disorders

Congenital heart disease (CHD) involves anatomic malformation(s) that develop in utero. There is a high risk for CHD with maternal diabetes, teratogen exposure, advanced maternal age, small for gestational age, very low and extremely low birthweights, prematurity, and chromosome anomalies. Signs of CHD do not always occur immediately after birth and are usually seen within the first two weeks of life. Cyanotic heart defects may not show signs until the ductus arteriosus closes. Cyanotic heart defects have decreased pulmonary blood flow, a right to left shunt, a right outflow obstruction from the heart is present, and there is cyanosis. General signs of cyanotic heart defects include right sided heart failure, hepatomegaly, metabolic acidosis, poor perfusion, hypoglycemia, a murmur may be present, prominent right ventricle and atria, and oligemic lung fields. Acyanotic heart defects may have signs including pulmonary symptoms of congestive heart failure, murmur, metabolic acidosis, hypoglycemia, cardiomegaly, and pulmonary edema. CHD may not be immediately diagnosed, although defects may be detected in utero with ultrasound. Testing may include electrocardiogram (ECG), hyperoxia test, and echocardiogram (Gardner et al., 2020; Maryniak, 2023).

Transposition of the great arteries (TGA), also known as transposition of the great vessels, is a cyanotic defect in which there is an inversion of parallel tubes in embryonic development, and the transposed arteries create two parallel circulations. In TGA, the aorta carries desaturated blood back to the systemic circulation and the pulmonary artery carries oxygenated blood back to the lungs (see Fig. 1.1). Survival occurs with a patent ductus arteriosus in addition to a communication at the atrial/ventricular level to allow oxygenated blood to reach the body. Management of TGA may include the use of prostaglandin immunoglobulin to maintain a patent ductus arteriosus (PDA), maintain and correct electrolytes, a balloon atrioseptostomy, and an arterial switch as the final repair (Gardner et al., 2020; Maryniak, 2023).

Tricuspid atresia is another cyanotic heart defect, which occurs when there is no development of the valve between right atrium and ventricle (see Fig. 1.2). Signs of tricuspid atresia depend on the presence and size of septal communication. A murmur may or may not be present. Management of tricuspid atresia may include prostaglandin E (PGE) administration to maintain an open ductus

Cardiac Disorders

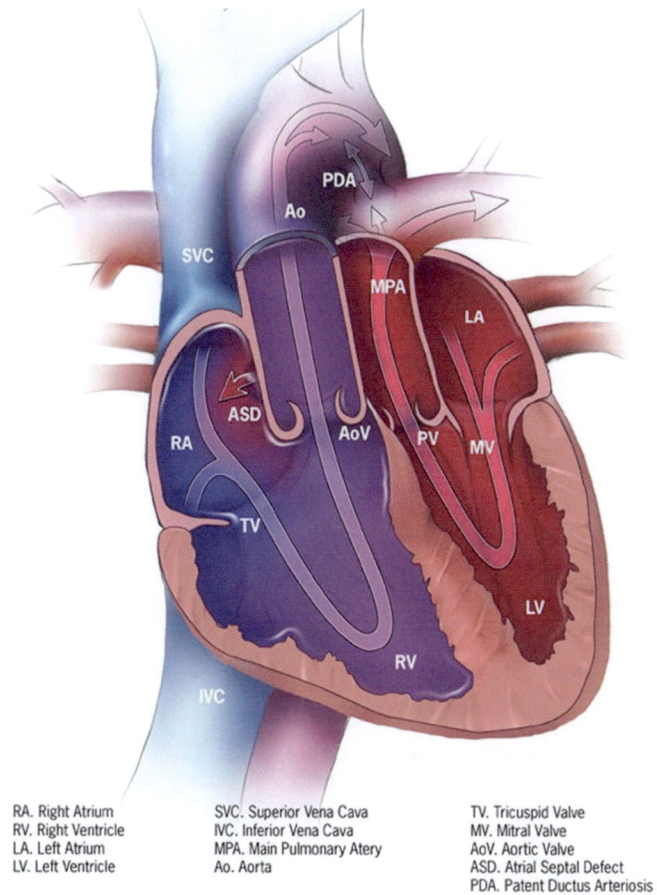

RA. Right Atrium	SVC. Superior Vena Cava	TV. Tricuspid Valve
RV. Right Ventricle	IVC. Inferior Vena Cava	MV. Mitral Valve
LA. Left Atrium	MPA. Main Pulmonary Atery	AoV. Aortic Valve
LV. Left Ventricle	Ao. Aorta	ASD. Atrial Septal Defect
		PDA. Patent Ductus Arteriosis

Fig. 1.1 Transposition of the great arteries. (Centers for Disease Control and Prevention, National Center on Birth Defects and Developmental Disabilities. https://www.cdc.gov/ncbddd/heartdefects/d-tga.html)

arteriosus, a surgical Blalock-Taussig (BT) shunt implant between the subclavian and pulmonary arteries, pulmonary artery banding, and a Fontan procedure, which is the corrective repair (Gardner et al., 2020; Maryniak, 2023).

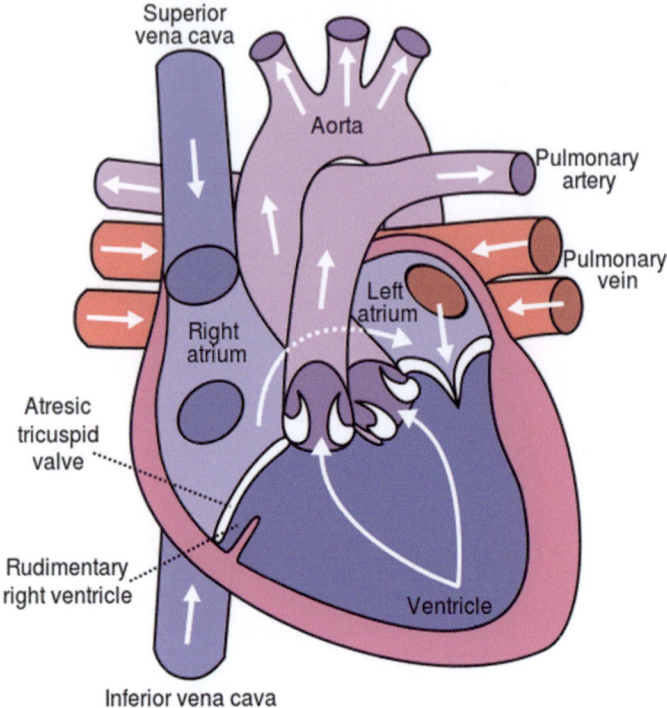

Fig. 1.2 Tricuspid atresia. (Centers for Disease Control and Prevention, National Center on Birth Defects and Developmental Disabilities. https://www.cdc.gov/ncbddd/heartdefects/tricuspid-atresia.html)

An additional cyanotic heart defect is tetralogy of Fallot, which actually has multiple defects (see Fig. 1.3). These defects are pulmonary atresia or stenosis, right ventricular hypertrophy, an overriding aorta, and a large ventricular septal defect (VSD). Tetralogy of Fallot may not be seen in the neonatal period if there is adequate mixing of oxygenated and unoxygenated blood and shunts for blood flow. Management of tetralogy of Fallot includes metabolic and volume management, use of PGE to maintain the patency of a PDA, a BT shunt, between subclavian and pulmonary arteries, and closure of the VSD with a patch (Gardner et al., 2020; Maryniak, 2023).

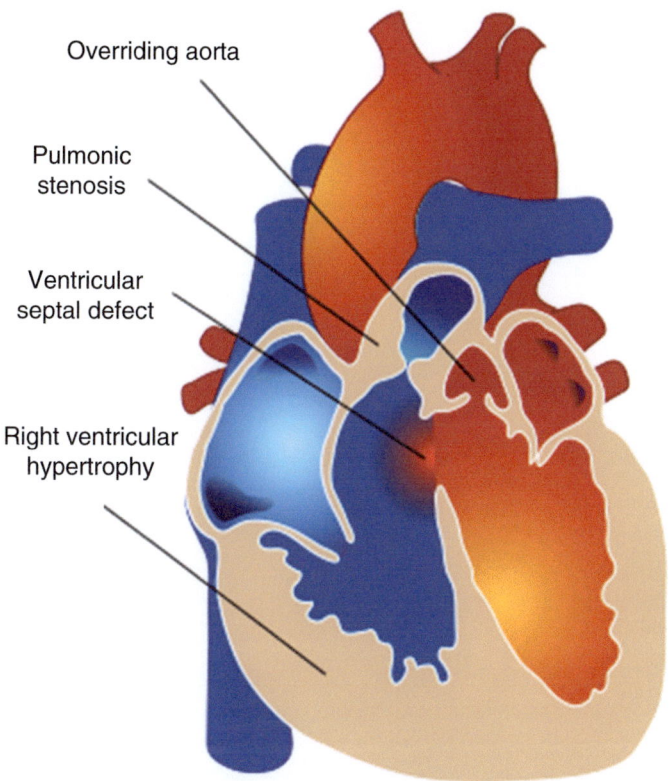

Fig. 1.3 Tetralogy of Fallot. (Centers for Disease Control and Prevention, National Center on Birth Defects and Developmental Disabilities. https://www.cdc.gov/ncbddd/heartdefects/tetralogyoffallot.html)

Another cyanotic heart defect is truncus arteriosus, where one artery forms both the pulmonary artery and the aorta in utero (see Fig. 1.4). With this condition, mixed blood is pumped to the body, and a VSD is almost always associated with truncus arteriosus. Management of truncus arteriosus includes PGE administration to maintain an open ductus arteriosus, treatment of congestive heart failure, creating a graft between the right ventricle and pulmonary artery, pulmonary artery banding, and closure of the VSD (Gardner et al., 2020; Maryniak, 2023).

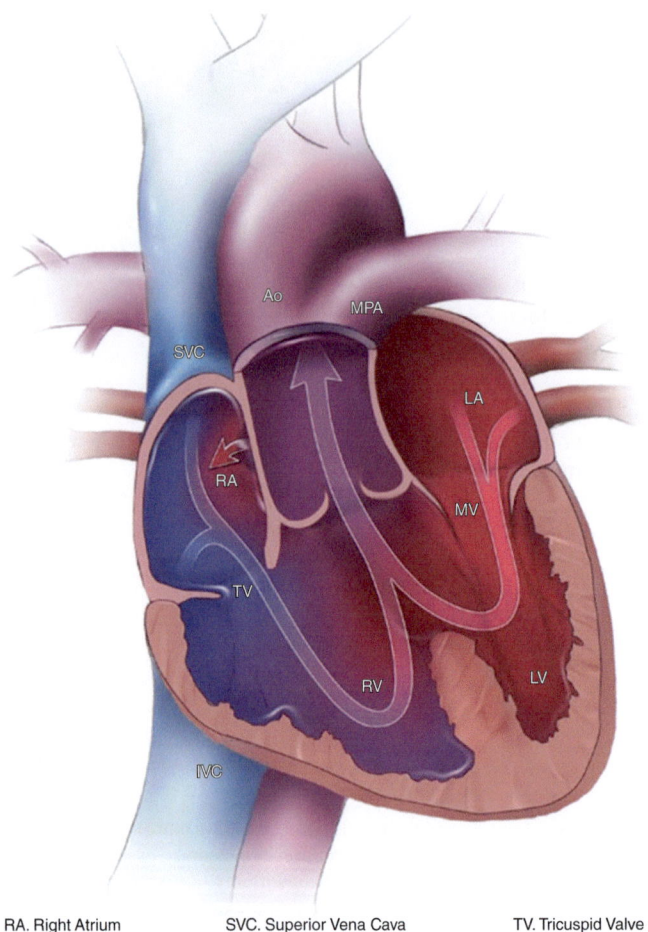

RA. Right Atrium
RV. Right Ventricle
LA. Left Atrium
LV. Left Ventricle

SVC. Superior Vena Cava
IVC. Inferior Vena Cava
MPA. Main Pulmonary Artery
Ao. Aorta

TV. Tricuspid Valve
MV. Mitral Valve

Fig. 1.4 Truncus arteriosus. (Centers for Disease Control and Prevention, National Center on Birth Defects and Developmental Disabilities. https://www.cdc.gov/ncbddd/heartdefects/truncusarteriosus.html)

Total anomalous pulmonary venous return (TAPVR) is another cyanotic heart defect where the pulmonary veins drain into the right atrium instead of the left atrium (see Fig. 1.5). Management

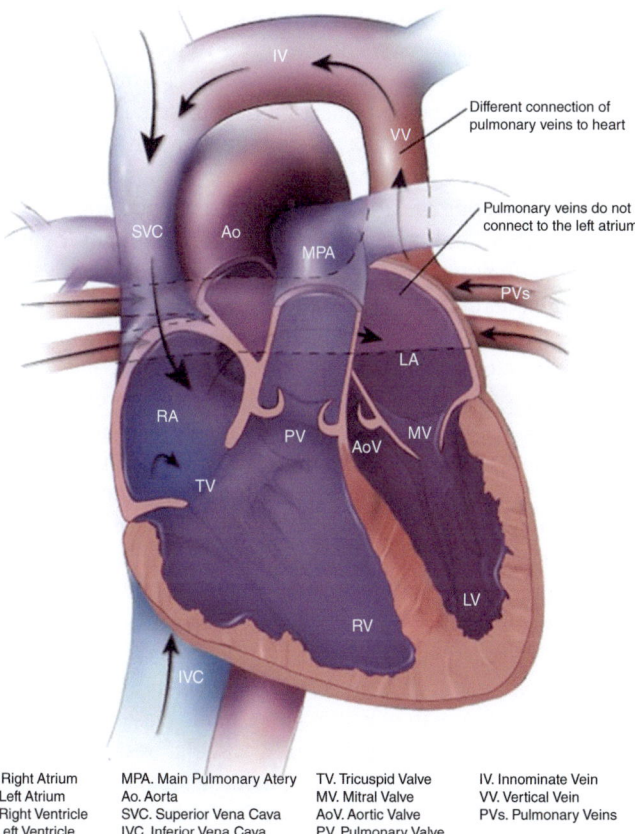

Fig. 1.5 Total anomalous pulmonary venous return. (Centers for Disease Control and Prevention, National Center on Birth Defects and Developmental Disabilities. https://www.cdc.gov/ncbddd/heartdefects/tapvr.html)

of TAPVR involves administration of PGE to maintain an open ductus arteriosus, create communication between the right and left sides of the heart to survive, closure of a PDA, and detachment of anomalous veins with transplantation to the left atrium (Gardner et al., 2020; Maryniak, 2023).

Pulmonary stenosis and pulmonary atresia are also cyanotic heart defects. Pulmonary stenosis refers to the narrowing of the pulmonary valve, while pulmonary atresia is a malformation of the valve. These conditions increase the pressure in the right side of the heart, causing right ventricular hypertrophy, and may have a VSD as well. Management of pulmonary atresia or stenosis includes correcting metabolic imbalances, maintaining a PDA by using PGE, an atrial septectomy, pulmonary valvotomy, right ventricular outflow tract reconstruction and patching, and a Fontan procedure (Gardner et al., 2020; Maryniak, 2023).

Patent ductus arteriosus (PDA) is a heart defect where the ductus fails to close, which is influenced by hypoxia and acidosis. The amount and direction of blood shunting through a PDA depends on peripheral and systemic vascular resistance, and the size of the PDA. Signs include murmur, widened pulse pressure, bounding or full pulses, fluctuations in oxygen requirements, and pulmonary congestion and edema. Management of patent ductus arteriosus includes fluid and nutrition management, indomethacin or ibuprofen to medically close the ductus, surgical ligation, and ventilation and cardiotropic support in severe cases (Gardner et al., 2020; Maryniak, 2023).

Persistent pulmonary hypertension (PPHN) happens when there isn't a normal increase in systemic vascular resistance (SVR) and decrease in pulmonary vascular resistance (PVR). After delivery, asphyxia, hypoxia, acidosis, and other complications causes an increase in PVR. A PDA with a right to left shunt also occurs with PPHN. Signs of PPHN may include murmur, oligemic lung fields, hypoxia, hypercarbia, acidosis, hypoglycemia, cyanosis, metabolic acidosis, and a difference between preductal and post ductal PaO_2. There are specific considerations for treating PPHN. Management of PPHN may include neutral thermal environment, minimal handling, vasopressors, sedation, carefully titrated oxygen, high frequency ventilation (HFV), nitric oxide

(NO), and extracorporeal membrane oxygenation (ECMO) (Gardner et al., 2020; Maryniak, 2023).

An atrial septal defect (ASD) occurs when there is a defect between the atria (see Fig. 1.6). Oxygenated blood shunts through ASD from left to right, and mixes with deoxygenated blood. ASD

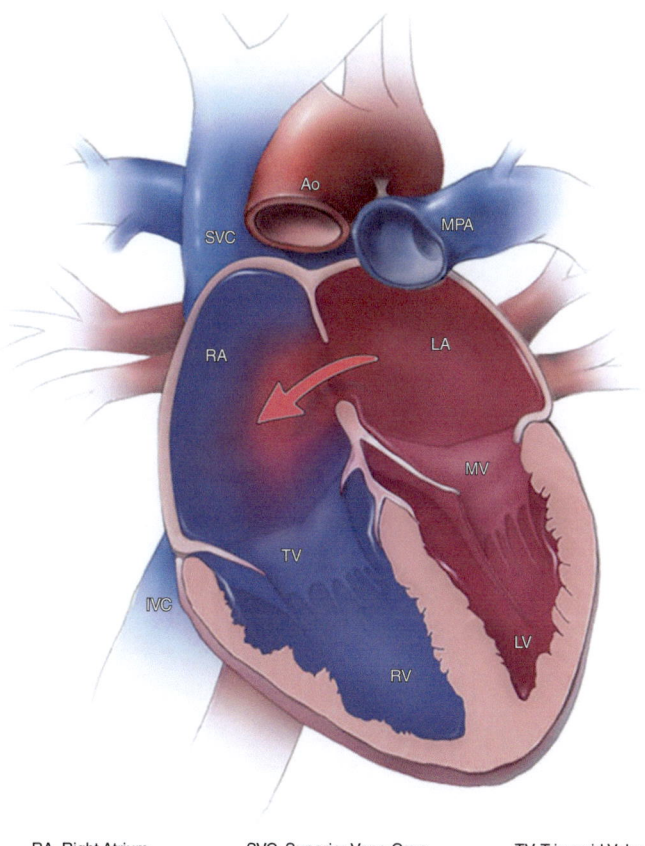

RA. Right Atrium
RV. Right Ventricle
LA. Left Atrium
LV. Left Ventricle

SVC. Superior Vena Cava
IVC. Inferior Vena Cava
MPA. Main Pulmonary Artery
Ao. Aorta

TV. Tricuspid Valve
MV. Mitral Valve

Fig. 1.6 Atrial septal defect. (Centers for Disease Control and Prevention, National Center on Birth Defects and Developmental Disabilities. https://www.cdc.gov/ncbddd/heartdefects/atrialseptaldefect.html)

has minor effects on circulatory status and is usually found with other heart defects. Neonates with ASD may be asymptomatic, have a murmur, dyspnea, or fatigue. ASDs generally close on their own, although a patch can be used or, rarely, surgical closure (Gardner et al., 2020; Maryniak, 2023).

A ventricular septal defect (VSD) is when there is a defect between the ventricles, with mixing of blood (see Fig. 1.7).

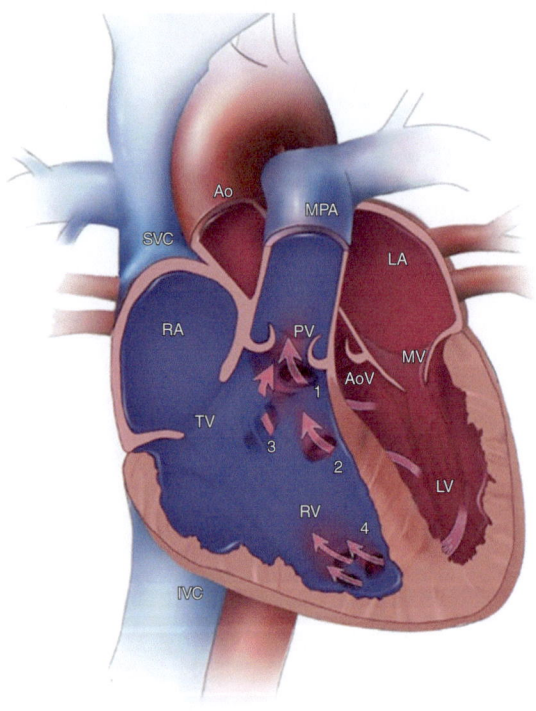

RA. Right Atrium	SVC. Superior Vena Cava	TV. Tricuspid Valve	1. Conoventricular, malaligned
RV. Right Ventricle	IVC. Inferior Vena Cava	MV. Mitral Valve	2. perimembranous
LA. Left Atrium	MPA. Main Pulmonary Artery	PV. Pulmonary Valve	3. inlet
LV. Left Ventricle	Ao. Aorta	AoV. Aortic Valve	4. muscular

Fig. 1.7 Ventricular septal defect. (Centers for Disease Control and Prevention, National Center on Birth Defects and Developmental Disabilities. https://www.cdc.gov/ncbddd/heartdefects/ventricularseptaldefect.html)

This may minimally impact circulation unless the VSD is large enough to cause congestive heart failure (CHF) from pulmonary over-circulation. Neonates with a VSD may be asymptomatic, may have a murmur, poor weight gain, and fatigue. The defect may close on its own without treatment. CHF may necessitate VSD repair through a patch or surgical closure (Gardner et al., 2020; Maryniak, 2023).

Coarctation of the aorta is the constriction or narrowing of the aorta, which may be pre- or post-ductal (see Fig. 1.8). A PDA is needed to maintain the systemic circulation as a result of diminished perfusion to body after the narrowing in the aorta. There is a difference in upper and lower limb perfusion, which is the main sign of coarctation, which may not be present until after the ductus has closed. Signs of coarctation of the aorta include differences in pulses and blood pressure of upper and lower extremities, pallor, dyspnea, irritability, and sweating. Management involves correcting the narrowing of the aorta through balloon angiography, stent placement, surgical reconstruction, or patching (Gardner et al., 2020; Maryniak, 2023).

Hypoplastic left heart syndrome (HLHS) is primarily due to the underdevelopment of the left ventricle and also includes other left-sided underdevelopment such as stenosis of the mitral and aortic valves, and hypoplasia of the aorta (see Fig. 1.9). A small left ventricle is unable to maintain adequate cardiac output, and, therefore, the PDA is the main source of systemic blood flow. There may not be symptoms initially if there is a PDA and a patent foramen ovale, and other signs may include pallor, cyanosis, dyspnea, weak pulse, and hypotension. HLHS is managed depending on the severity and associated morbidities, including heart transplant or a three-stage surgery, with use of PGE to maintain ductus prior to surgery. In some cases palliative care may be the only option (Gardner et al., 2020; Maryniak, 2023).

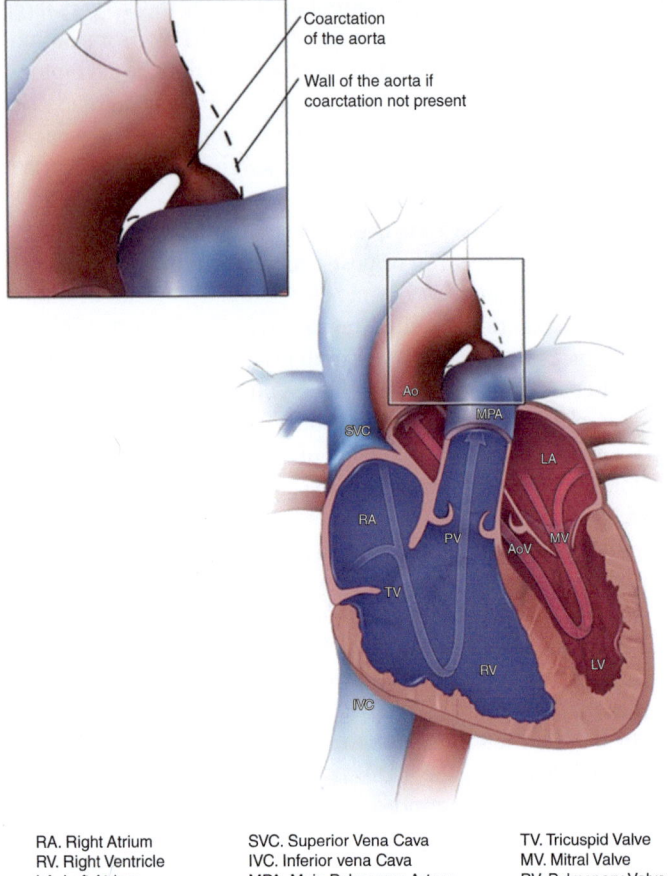

RA. Right Atrium	SVC. Superior Vena Cava	TV. Tricuspid Valve
RV. Right Ventricle	IVC. Inferior vena Cava	MV. Mitral Valve
LA. Left Atrium	MPA. Main Pulmonary Artery	PV. Pulmonary Valve
LV. Left Ventricle	Ao. Aorta	AoV. Aortic Valve

Fig. 1.8 Coarctation of the aorta. (Centers for Disease Control and Prevention, National Center on Birth Defects and Developmental Disabilities https://www.cdc.gov/ncbddd/heartdefects/coarctationofaorta.html)

Cardiac Disorders

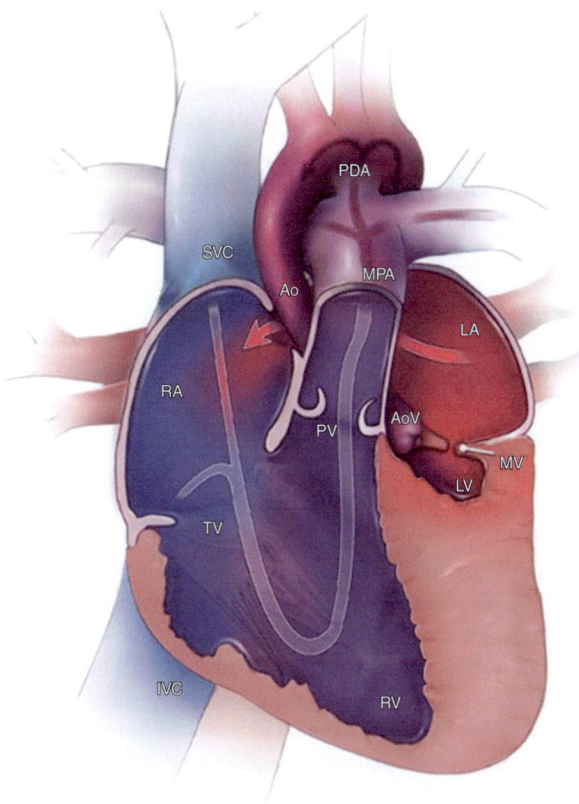

RA. Right Atrium
RV. Right Ventricle
LA. Left Atrium
LV. Left Ventricle

SVC. Superior Vena Cava
IVC. Inferior Vena Cava
MPA. Main Pulmonary Artery
Ao. Aorta
PDA. Patent Ductus Arteriosis

TV. Tricuspid Valve
MV. Mitral Valve
PV. Pulmonary Valve
AoV. Aortic Valve

Fig. 1.9 Hypoplastic left heart syndrome. (Centers for Disease Control and Prevention, National Center on Birth Defects and Developmental Disabilities https://www.cdc.gov/ncbddd/heartdefects/hlhs.html)

Toddlers

Children aged one to three years are considered toddlers. During this time period, many physical skills are developed, such as walking, running, climbing, throwing and dropping toys, stacking blocks, and developing certain fine motor skills. Toddlers can achieve control of the bladder and bowel. They are active and energetic and require close monitoring to ensure safety (Maryniak, 2019).

According to Erikson, the stage of development for toddlers is autonomy versus shame and doubt. As autonomy develops for a toddler, they begin to establish a central identity, depend less on the parents or primary caregivers, and accept brief separation from the parents or caregiver. Shame and doubt can develop if the toddler does not develop autonomy, which can be demonstrated as a low tolerance for frustration, or lack of self-confidence (Balasundaram & Avulakunta, 2023).

It is important to have close contact between toddlers and parents or caregivers, and nurses can assist parents or caregivers to set safe rules, limits, and boundaries. Autonomy development can be assisted by allowing the toddler to make small choices about medical procedures and examinations (as appropriate), and giving simple explanations about medical procedures before beginning. Using a firm, direct approach, emphasizing what actions will require the toddler's cooperation, and encouraging parents or caregivers to participate in procedures with the toddler will help develop good relationships (Maryniak, 2019).

Toddlers have high energy, are impulsive, and are natural explorers but cannot recognize danger and may end up in unsafe situations without close monitoring. Increased autonomy also increases risks of accidents and injuries, such as choking or poisoning. It is important to keep medications, small objects, and chemicals out of their reach.

Toddlers can learn about and participate in certain portions of their own care. Toddlers learn through discovery and imitation, and as they progress, their verbal skills also advance, with improved vocabulary. They can comprehend explanations which are concrete and they can also follow simple commands. The sense of time for toddlers does not go beyond what is immediately happening, and space does not go beyond what they can see, creating short attention spans. It is important to use short, simple, concrete explanations with words the toddler can understand, and give one direction at a time. Use visuals to demonstrate, such as books, dolls, and toys, and give the toddler praise when they show correct behavior (Maryniak, 2019).

Pneumonia

Worldwide, pneumonia is a leading cause of morbidity and mortality of children less than five years old. The main source of pneumonia is commonly respiratory viruses, and for toddlers the most common pathogens include *Streptococcus pneumoniae* and *Haemophilus influenzae* (Ebeledike & Ahmad, 2023). Pneumonia occurs from a pathogen invading the lower respiratory tract, creating infection. This infection causes inflammation, injury, or death of the epithelium and alveoli, creating exudate, which impairs oxygenation. Signs and symptoms of pneumonia include fever, tachypnea, and decreased oxygenation as well as decreased breath sounds, rales, rhonchi, or crackles on auscultation (Ebeledike & Ahmad, 2023).

Rapid nasopharyngeal testing should be done for influenza, respiratory syncytial virus, and COVID prior to performing imaging to avoid unnecessary exposure to radiation. History and physical examination along with blood work can help determine the cause of the infection. Pneumonia is confirmed with a chest x-ray. Management includes oxygen support, fluids, and antipyretics. Antibiotics are used empirically only if bacterial infection is suspected. For toddlers, if *Streptococcus pneumoniae* is suspected, treatment includes amoxicillin or other beta-lactam antibiotics. Potential complications of pneumonia in the pediatric patient include empyema, pleural effusion, lung abscess, and sepsis (Ebeledike & Ahmad, 2023).

Bronchitis

Acute bronchitis creates inflammation of the trachea, bronchi, and bronchioles, and is usually associated with lower respiratory tract infections from viruses in pediatric patients. Acute bronchitis generally resolves within two weeks, but recurrent inflammation can cause chronic bronchitis. Chronic bronchitis is also associated with cystic fibrosis, asthma, foreign bodies, or airway irritants (Carolan, 2023).

The main symptoms of bronchitis include cough and nasal discharge. Dyspnea may also be present, as well as malaise, chills, sore throat, mild fever, and myalgia. Laboratory workup may include serum C-reactive protein, respiratory culture, and rapid diagnostic studies to determine the source of pathogen. Testing for asthma, cystic fibrosis, and immunodeficiencies may also be done. Chest x-rays, if performed, are generally normal. Management includes oxygenation and hydration, use of antipyretics as warranted, and management of underlying causes of bronchitis (Carolan, 2023).

Asthma

Asthma involves interactions among inflammatory and resident airway cells, creating inflammation in airways, intermittent obstruction of airflow, and bronchial hyperresponsiveness. In children under the age of six, including toddlers, sporadic symptoms can occur which may resolve in childhood. Other children can develop chronic asthma which persists into adulthood. There are genetic and environmental risk factors which increase the likelihood of developing asthma. In addition to genetic markers, risk factors include maternal smoking in pregnancy, prematurity, male gender, exposure to allergens, and obesity (Lizzo et al., 2024).

The most prominent symptoms of asthma are cough and wheezing. Coughing tends to worsen at night. Other symptoms may include nasal discharge, shortness of breath, dyspnea, fatigue, disrupted sleep, tachypnea, hypoxia, prolonged expiratory phase, and retractions or use of accessory muscles. Spirometry is often used to confirm diagnosis. If chest x-ray is performed, results often show hyperinflated lungs. Acute asthma management depends on the severity, and short-acting β-agonists such as albuterol is used for symptoms, usually via nebulizer. Glucocorticoids, inhaled short-acting muscarinic antagonists, and β-agonists such as epinephrine and terbutaline may also be used in severe exacerbations. Supplemental oxygen may also be necessary (Lizzo et al., 2024).

Acute Respiratory Failure

Toddlers can also be hospitalized for acute respiratory failure from infections, diseases, or disorders, similar to infants. Toddlers with asthma, pneumonia, or other respiratory illness can show signs of impending respiratory failure if they continue to decompensate despite treatment, such as cyanosis, decreased mental status, continued low oxygen saturation, respiratory distress and increased work of breathing, and respiratory acidosis (Lizzo et al., 2024). Symptoms and management of acute respiratory failure are described above in the section on infants.

Fluid and Electrolyte Imbalance

Electrolyte imbalances can occur in children leading to hospitalizations. Sodium and potassium imbalances will be discussed. Hyponatremia is the most common imbalance in toddlers, which is considered as a serum sodium level of less than 135 mmol/L (Zieg et al., 2024). Extracellular fluid depletion and subsequent sodium loss from dehydration through vomiting, diarrhea, or other conditions is a common cause of hyponatremia. Symptoms of hyponatremia include headache, lethargy, altered level of consciousness, confusion, nausea, vomiting, and in severe cases seizures, coma, and respiratory and cardiac arrest. Management of hyponatremia includes incremental sodium replacement with frequent monitoring to avoid overcorrection. Underlying conditions and volume status are also managed (Zieg et al., 2024).

Hypernatremia can also occur with toddlers, considered as a serum sodium level of greater than 145 mmol/L. Viral gastroenteritis is a common cause of hypernatremia (Zieg et al., 2024). Symptoms of hypernatremia are fever, irritability, and weakness, and when severe, lethargy, altered mental status, neurological defects, coma, seizures, and death may occur. Management includes initial isotonic solutions intravenously, and then solutions with higher free water content to correct hypernatremia. Monitoring of sodium levels is essential to prevent a rapid decline in sodium (Zieg et al., 2024).

Although more common in children older than four years of age, imbalances in potassium can also occur in toddlers. Hypokalemia is considered at serum potassium levels less than 3.5 mmol/L. Fluid loss through vomiting, diarrhea, or malabsorption is a common cause of hypokalemia. Renal dysfunction can also create potassium imbalance. Symptoms of hypokalemia may include fatigue, weakness, confusion, nausea, vomiting, and diarrhea. Severe symptoms include paralysis, respiratory failure, and arrhythmias such as ST depression and PR and QT prolongation. Oral potassium replacement is the recommended management of hypokalemia. Monitoring blood glucose levels is also needed, as high glucose can stimulate insulin, which further worsens hypokalemia (Zieg et al., 2024).

Hyperkalemia is when a serum potassium level is greater than 5.5 mmol/L, and is usually the result of kidney disease or acute kidney injury in children. Diabetic ketoacidosis can also cause hyperkalemia (Zieg et al., 2024). Symptoms include weakness, muscular paralysis, respiratory failure, and ECG changes such as peaked T waves, prolonged QRS complexes, and flattened P waves. Severe hyperkalemia may also cause atrioventricular block, ventricular tachycardia or fibrillation, and asystole. Management of hyperkalemia is based on severity, and includes calcium chloride or calcium gluconate and dextrose with insulin infusion. Acidosis, if present, also needs to be corrected. Close monitoring of electrolytes including potassium, sodium, calcium, and glucose is needed (Zieg et al., 2024).

Infections

Common skin and soft tissue infections that result in hospitalizations for toddlers include cellulitis, abscesses, bullous impetigo, and dermatitis with superinfection. Bacterial infections with or without skin trauma are most common, followed by viral and fungal pathogens (Brigadoi et al., 2024). Cellulitis presents as skin that is red, warm to touch, swollen, and painful (see Fig. 1.10). Other symptoms may include fever, malaise, chills, and red streaking of the area (Herchline, 2024). Skin abscesses can also occur from pathogen invasion, resulting in a pocket of purulent material, pain, swelling, and redness (Brigadoi et al., 2024). Bullous impetigo results from bacterial infection, with *Staphylococcal Aureus* being the most common source (see Fig. 1.11). Bullous impetigo presents as superficial fragile bullae that can involve small or large lesions, generally occurring on the face, extremities, trunk, buttocks, and perineal areas. The lesions occur rapidly, rupture spontaneously, and then drain, and can spread locally. The lesions can

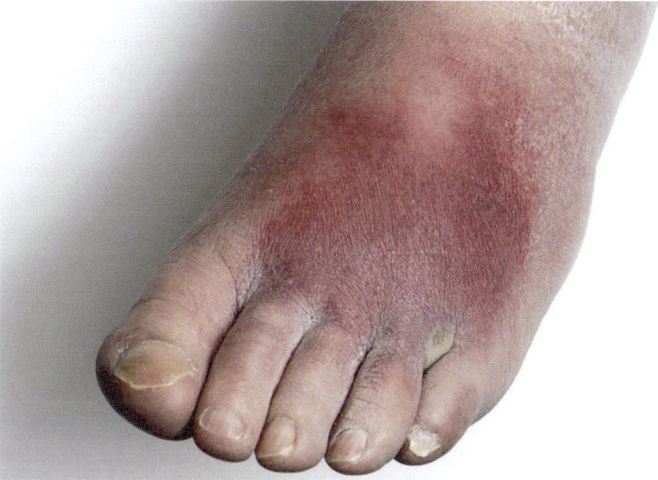

Fig. 1.10 Cellulitis. (Cellulitis: Image retrieved from https://www.nhs.uk/conditions/cellulitis/)

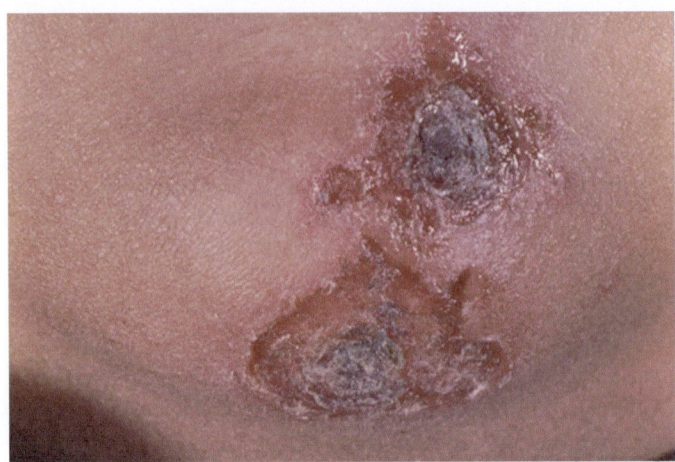

Fig. 1.11 Bullous impetigo. (Bullous impetigo: Image retrieved from Impetigo—NHS)

also superinfect other skin conditions, such as eczema and dermatitis. Fever, diarrhea, and weakness may also occur with bullous impetigo (Moon, 2023). Bacterial infection management in hospital involves intravenous antibiotics based upon the pathogen. Treatment is focused on symptoms, including pain and fluid management (Brigadoi et al., 2024).

Gastrointestinal infections can also be a reason for admission of toddlers to acute care hospitals. Rotavirus is the most common pathogen up to 24 months of age, with *Shigella* commonly causing gastroenteritis after 24 months of age (Rivera-Dominguez & Ward, 2023). Signs and symptoms may include fever (although not always present), nausea, vomiting, watery diarrhea, and abdominal pain. Management of gastroenteritis in the toddler focuses on rehydration as discussed in the infant section. Rehydration may include oral or IV fluids. Antiemetics may be administered, but it is not recommended to provide antidiarrheal medications. Testing should be done to determine the causative pathogen, and antibiotics are only warranted when gastroenteritis is bacterial (Rivera-Dominguez & Ward, 2023).

Seizures and Epilepsy

Seizures occur from abnormal neuronal activity that create signs and symptoms from involuntary muscle activity. The risk factors for seizures in a pediatric patient include family history, fever, infections, central nervous system comorbidities, maternal alcohol or tobacco abuse during pregnancy, and prematurity (Minardi et al., 2019). Seizures are caused by various factors, including structural changes in the brain, genetic, infectious, metabolic, and immune influences, or of unknown etiology. Younger children, including toddlers, commonly have seizures associated with fever or infections. Seizures are diagnosed by electroencephalogram (EEG). Epilepsy is considered as two unprovoked seizures occurred greater than 24 hours apart, or one unprovoked seizure and a probability of further seizures over the next ten years, or a diagnosis of epilepsy syndrome (Minardi et al., 2019). With focal seizures, the patient may be awake or have impaired consciousness, have non-motor components such as cognitive, behavioral, and sensory deficits, and motor components such as tonic or clonic movements that may be focal or bilateral. Generalized seizures impair consciousness and are associated with generalized motor symptoms such as tonic, clonic, or both (Minardi et al., 2019). Management of seizures includes providing safety for the patient during seizure episodes, treating the cause, and preventing further seizures through use of anti-epileptic medications (Minardi et al., 2019).

Pediatric Cancer

Pediatric cancer can occur at any age in childhood. Toddlers have higher incidence of leukemia and non-central nervous system (CNS) embryonal cancer, in addition to cancer of the CNS, bone cancer, lymphomas, and other solid tumors (Lupo & Spector, 2020). For the purpose of this section, non-CNS cancers (neuroblastoma, nephroblastoma) will be explored.

Although there is variation in the literature, some risk factors for developing various pediatric cancers have been identified. Exposures in utero to smoking, environmental carcinogens, alcohol, and radiation are risk factors. Advanced maternal age, birth defects, high or low birthweight, and gestational age can also be associated with pediatric cancers. Chemical and radiation exposure in childhood as well as second-hand smoke are also risk factors. Breastfeeding and use of maternal vitamins are inversely related to pediatric cancer (Lupo & Spector, 2020).

Neuroblastomas are the most common form of non-CNS pediatric embryonal cancer (Mahapatra & Challagundla, 2023). Most neuroblastomas occur in the adrenal glands, but can also present in the neck, chest, abdomen, or pelvis. Patients may be asymptomatic or have signs and symptoms related to the site of the tumor. These can include fever, fatigue, weight loss, paralysis, chronic diarrhea, pain, and changes in gait. Neuroblastomas can spread to the bone and bone marrow, lymph nodes, and lungs (Mahapatra & Challagundla, 2023).

Complete blood count (CBC), liver and renal panels, electrolytes, and lactate can be affected, and diagnosis of neuroblastoma is confirmed through histology and diagnostic imaging, including magnetic resonance imaging (MRI) and computed tomography (CT) (Mahapatra & Challagundla, 2023).

Neuroblastoma management depends on the size, location, grade of the tumor, and stage of cancer. Options for treatment include surgical resection, chemotherapy, radiation therapy, stem cell transplantation, and immunotherapy, in addition to patient monitoring (Mahapatra & Challagundla, 2023).

A nephroblastoma is also known as Wilms tumor and is the most common pediatric renal cancer and is usually found in children younger than five (Leslie et al., 2023). Genetic abnormalities may be involved in developing nephroblastoma. Many time patients have an asymptomatic abdominal mass but may also display symptoms of pain, hematuria, urinary tract infection, varicocele, blood pressure changes (either hypotension or hypertension), fever, anemia, and dyspnea (Leslie et al., 2023).

Diagnostic testing includes CBC, electrolytes, renal panel, urinalysis, and coagulation studies. Genetic testing may be performed. Imaging includes renal ultrasound, chest x-ray, and abdominal and chest CT. Histology can provide confirmation (Leslie et al., 2023).

Management of nephroblastoma does depend on staging, and includes surgical removal of the affected kidney and chemotherapy. Radiation may also be done post-surgery. Bilateral nephrectomy may be warranted (Leslie et al., 2023).

Pre-school Aged Children

Pre-school aged children, or preschoolers, are between ages three and five years old. Fine motor skills and dexterity are improved, such as the abilities to walk on their tiptoes, stand on one foot, and hop, and they can dress and feed themselves. Verbal skills greatly improve with increased vocabulary to about 1000 words and four-to-six-word sentences. Preschoolers are able to reason logically, can use abstract thought, and are able to tell the difference between right and wrong. They can maintain attention for longer periods. Stories are important, and can assist the preschooler with learning, and they can also tell their own stories (Maryniak, 2019).

Erikson's stage of development for preschoolers is initiative versus guilt. Achieving initiative for preschoolers can improve self-confidence and they can act with intention and reason. Guilt may be demonstrated by fear of punishment, which can decrease their ability to act with purpose and direction (Balasundaram & Avulakunta, 2023).

Preschoolers need acknowledgement and encouragement of their physical accomplishments. Rewarding appropriate behavior with praise is important. Nurses should provide correct, age-appropriate information to the preschooler, such as explaining healthcare issues clearly, and describing what will be done in a firm and direct manner. Preschoolers are afraid of injury, and disease can be very upsetting. It is important to be honest if something will hurt, such as a procedure, but also emphasize that it will not hurt for long. Nurses can use toys, games, dolls, and books to demonstrate, and also provide distractions, such as talking, singing, and other activities. The preschooler's increasing independence can be fostered by providing choices and allowing them to control their environment as much as possible.

Preschoolers still have an inadequate ability to recognize danger and require close supervision. Limits, boundaries, and rules must still be clearly established. The preschooler can participate in education and can be encouraged to ask questions and discuss their feelings and fears. Play with other children should be facilitated, and the preschooler should be allowed to maintain comforting routines as much as possible. The imagination of preschoolers increases, and they learn through exploring, discovering, and asking questions. The preschooler may be provided with more detailed healthcare information. Explanations of unfamiliar objects should be given along with the use of correct terminology (Maryniak, 2019).

Infections

Like toddlers, preschoolers can also have skin and soft tissue infections that result in hospitalizations, such as cellulitis, abscesses (see Fig. 1.12), bullous impetigo, and dermatitis with superinfection (see Fig. 1.13). They can also be admitted with gastroenteritis. For further descriptions and management of these conditions, refer to the section on toddlers above.

Respiratory Illnesses

Upper respiratory tract infections are a common reason of hospitalization of the preschooler. Rhinovirus is the most frequently seen cause of upper respiratory infections, including the common cold, with a peak period seen in autumn. The rhinovirus has multiple serotypes, and symptoms may develop within 12 hours of exposure, persisting for up to three weeks (Thomas & Bomar,

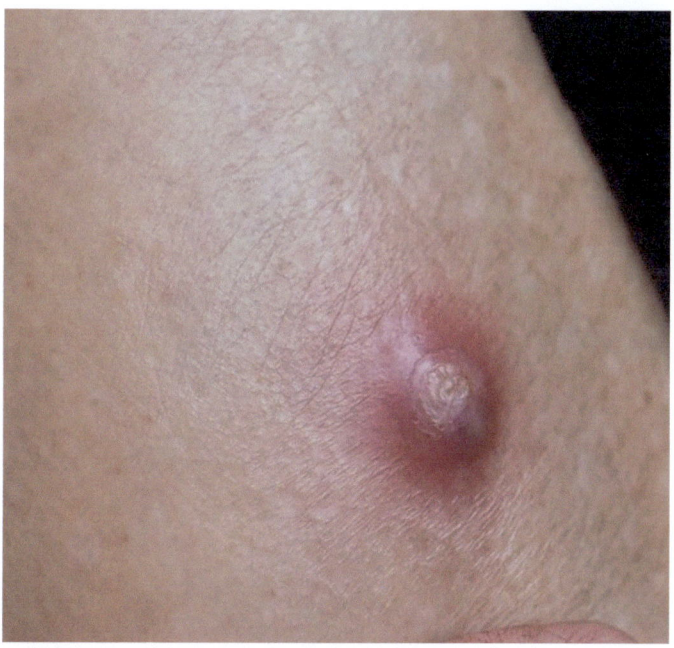

Fig. 1.12 Skin abscess. (Skin abscess: Image retrieved from https://www.nhs.uk/conditions/skin-abscess/)

2023). Signs and symptoms can include cough, rhinorrhea, sore throat, congestion, sneezing, low-grade fever, malaise, and myalgia. Management of rhinovirus is supportive, focusing on treating symptoms. Cough suppressants are not recommended for preschoolers. Fluids, rest, and management of any fever is recommended (Thomas & Bomar, 2023).

As previously discussed, pneumonia is a leading cause of morbidity and mortality of children under five years of age globally. The main source of pneumonia is commonly respiratory viruses, and for preschoolers the most common pathogens include *Haemophilus influenzae* B followed by *Streptococcus pneumoniae* (Ebeledike & Ahmad, 2023). For more detail on pneumonia, refer to the section on toddlers.

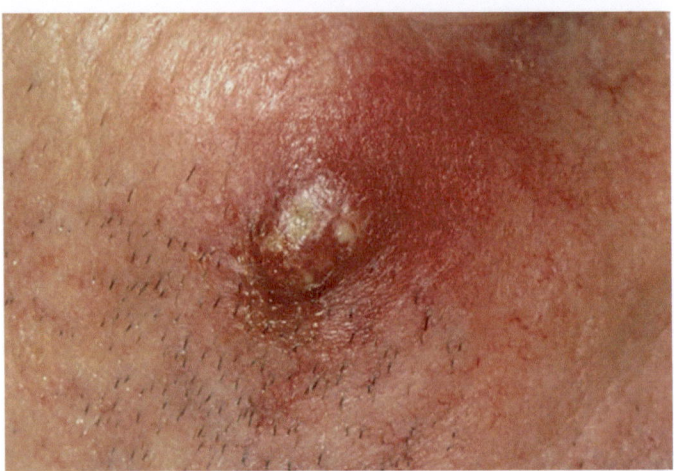

Fig. 1.13 Atopic dermatitis with superinfection. (Atopic dermatitis with superinfection: Image retrieved from https://www.nhs.uk/conditions/staphylococcal-infections/)

Influenza has four main types, with influenza A and B the common causes in the human population. Each strain also has subtypes. The transmission of influenza can occur prior to patients being symptomatic, and can continue to be contagious up to a week after symptoms resolve (Boktor & Hafner, 2023). Influenza can affect the upper and lower respiratory tract, and symptoms typically include rhinorrhea, high fever, cough, sore throat, headache, and myalgia. Patients who were vaccinated for influenza tend to have milder symptoms. Nucleic acid detection such as through polymerase chain reaction (PCR) testing confirms the influenza diagnosis. Supportive care is used with influenza, although antivirals may be used in some cases (Boktor & Hafner, 2023).

Another common respiratory illness seen in pediatric patients under the age of five is croup. The most frequent cause of croup is the parainfluenza virus, although other viral and bacterial pathogens may also be responsible (Sizar & Carr, 2023). Croup involves swelling of the larynx, trachea, and large bronchi due to infiltration of white blood cells, which causes partial airway obstruction.

Typical signs and symptoms are barking cough, stridor, and low-grade fever, generally lasting up to seven days. Management of croup may include dexamethasone, nebulized epinephrine, and oxygen (Sizar & Carr, 2023).

As mentioned in the toddler section, children under the age of six, including preschoolers, can develop intermittent asthma which resolve in childhood. Acute bronchitis can also be seen in this pediatric population. For further discussion on asthma, bronchitis, and management of these illnesses, refer to the section on toddlers above.

Pediatric Cancer

As previously discussed, pediatric cancer can occur at any age in childhood. Preschoolers have higher incidence of leukemia, followed by CNS tumors and non-CNS embryonal cancer. Other cancers include bone cancer, lymphomas, and other solid tumors (Lupo & Spector, 2020). For the purpose of this section, CNS tumors and leukemias will be discussed.

CNS tumors include diffuse low-grade gliomas (LGGs), high-grade gliomas (HGGs), ependymomas, and embryonal tumors. LGGs are the most common type of CNS tumor, making up about one-third of pediatric brain tumors. Although HGGs only account for about 10% of pediatric brain tumors, they are associated with poor outcomes. Ependymal tumors are up to 10% and embryonal tumors are approximately 20% of CNS tumors in children. Management of CNS tumors include resection, if possible, chemotherapy, and radiation therapy (Damodharan & Puccetti, 2023).

There are different types of leukemias, including acute lymphocytic (or lymphoblastic) leukemia (ALL), which makes up about 75% of pediatric leukemia, and acute myeloid (or myelogenous) leukemia (AML). Chronic myeloid leukemia (CML) and chronic lymphocytic leukemia (CLL) are the other two types, which are rare in pediatric patients (American Cancer Society, 2025).

ALL is a malignancy that causes uncontrolled spread of abnormal immature T or B lymphoblasts, replacing bone marrow and other lymph organ elements. Risk factors for ALL include male gender, Caucasian, genetic anomalies, and environmental exposures to radiation, chemotherapy, and benzene (Puckett & Chan, 2023). Signs and symptoms of ALL include palpable liver and spleen, pallor, fever, night sweats, weakness, bruising, lymphadenopathy, weakness, weight loss, dyspnea, myalgia or bone pain, and oliguria. Diagnosis and staging is done with CBC, biopsy, and CT scan of the abdomen and pelvis. Chemotherapy is the treatment of choice for ALL (Puckett & Chan, 2023).

AML if a fast-progressing myeloid neoplasm with clonal expansion of immature blasts in the blood and bone marrow. This can cause rapid bone marrow failure and depletion of red blood cells and platelets (Vakiti et al., 2024). Signs and symptoms of AML occur rapidly and include weakness, fatigue, headaches, recurrent infections, anemia, bruising, excessive bleeding, and shortness of breath. Management of AML is chemotherapy and stem cell transplantation (Vakiti et al., 2024).

Seizures and Epilepsy

Seizures and epilepsy can occur throughout childhood, including during the preschooler period. Refer to the section on toddlers for discussion of these conditions and management.

Diabetes

Diabetes mellitus, or just diabetes, is a chronic illness from defects in insulin production, insulin action, or both (Sapra & Bhandari, 2023). The main types of diabetes that affect pediatric patients are type 1 and type 2. Patients with diabetes may be asymptomatic, but typical symptoms include polyuria, polydipsia, polyphagia, weight loss, dehydration, fatigue, nausea, and vomiting. Diabetes is diagnosed with a fasting blood glucose of greater than or equal to 126 mg/dL, an A1C of 6.5% or higher, or a combination of both.

Type 1 diabetes is an auto-immune disease in which the body's immune system attacks and destroys the insulin-producing beta cells in the pancreas, resulting in the need for exogenous insulin to survive. This form of diabetes usually strikes children and young adults, although disease onset can occur at any age. Risk factors for type 1 diabetes may be autoimmune, genetic, or environmental (Sapra & Bhandari, 2023). Management of type 1 diabetes is the requirement of exogenous insulin as well as lifestyle changes of glucose monitoring, exercise, and dietary changes (Sapra & Bhandari, 2023).

Type 2 diabetes usually begins as insulin resistance, and as the need for insulin rises, the pancreas loses its ability to effectively produce it. Type 2 diabetes in children is associated with obesity, family history of diabetes, impaired glucose metabolism, physical inactivity, and race and ethnicity. There are high risks for type 2 diabetes in African Americans, Hispanic Americans, American Indians, and some Asian Americans, native Hawaiians, or other Pacific Islanders. Management of type 2 diabetes includes lifestyle changes such as exercise, diet, and monitoring blood glucose. Oral hypoglycemic medications can be used, with metformin considered the first line (Sapra & Bhandari, 2023).

Diabetic ketoacidosis (DKA) occurs from lack of insulin, which prevents metabolism of glucose. The body begins utilizing fat for fuel, and there is a buildup of ketones as a result of fat breakdown. The liver attempts to compensate by producing more glucose, causing further hyperglycemia (El-Mohandes et al., 2023). DKA is associated with infection, stress, cardiovascular disease, new onset, and missed insulin doses. DKA is typically seen in patients with type 1 diabetes, and can be associated with the initial diagnosis of diabetes. Although unusual, type 2 diabetics can also develop DKA. Symptoms of DKA are polyuria, polydipsia, polyphagia, weakness, fatigue, nausea, vomiting, Kussmaul breathing, coma, and fruity breath odor. DKA management includes IV hydration, IV insulin, correction of acidosis and hypokalemia as needed, and frequent monitoring of blood glucose, blood urea nitrogen, creatinine, sodium, potassium, and bicarbonate levels (El-Mohandes et al., 2023).

Hyperosmolar hyperglycemic state (HHS) is when blood glucose rises to dangerously high levels without ketones in the urine. Pediatric HHS is usually caused by infections (Adeyinka & Kondamudi, 2023). Signs and symptoms of HHS include fatigue, confusion, weakness, vision changes, high fever, dehydration, extreme thirst, and dry skin that is warm to touch. Management of HHS is IV hydration, IV insulin, and correction of electrolytes as needed (Adeyinka & Kondamudi, 2023).

School-Aged Children

Children between the ages of six and twelve years are considered school-aged. The physical growth of school-aged children is relatively slow until puberty, which then causes a rapid increase in growth. The puberty onset varies among children and may not occur until the adolescent stage. School-aged children are very active; there is an increase in neuromuscular skills, improved balance, and gain in muscular strength. Cause and effect can be understood, and logic and deductive reasoning is used to arrive at conclusions. Reading, writing, and mathematic skills are developed. School-aged children can understand past, present, future, and the finality of death (Maryniak, 2019).

The stage of development according to Erikson for school-aged children is industry versus inferiority. Children who develop industry can show competency, achievement, and self-confidence. Signs of inferiority, on the other hand, have feelings of inadequacy and fear of failing to meet the expectations of others (Balasundaram & Avulakunta, 2023).

School-aged children need reassurance about their physical changes, especially as they enter puberty, and need honest answers to questions about physical sexual characteristics. They need opportunities for making decisions and providing self-care, encouraging questions and verbalization of feelings, and upholding the need for privacy. It is also important to recognize the child's achievements. If children have a prolonged hospitalization, they should have schooling provided, and be encouraged to have peer contact.

School-aged children are enthusiastic learners, and they love to share their knowledge. They still have a limited understanding of anatomy, bodily functions, and illness, but should be provided with more complete healthcare information. Medical procedures should be explained in straightforward terms with the use of the correct terminology. School-aged children should be allowed to examine medical equipment prior to use. The child's attention span also needs to be considered (Maryniak, 2019).

Diabetes

Like preschoolers, school-aged children can also be admitted to hospital with type 1 or type 2 diabetes, DKA, or HHS. These can be a primary diagnosis or comorbidity. For further discussion and management, refer to the section on preschoolers above.

Pediatric Cancer

In the school-aged child, all pediatric cancers can be seen, including leukemia, non-CNS embryonal cancer, CNS tumors, bone cancer, lymphomas, and other solid tumors (Lupo & Spector, 2020). For the purpose of this section, the bone cancer osteosarcoma will be reviewed.

Primary bone cancer makes up about 5% of malignant pediatric cancers. Risk factors for bone cancer include genetic abnormalities, previous radiation therapy, and benign conditions such as Paget disease. Over half of the pediatric bone cancer in school-aged children is comprised of osteosarcomas (Pullan & Lotfollahzadeh, 2024). Osteosarcoma is tumor that can develop in any bone that quickly becomes malignant. These tumors are most common near the metaphysis of long bones in children, such as distal femur, proximal tibia, and proximal humerus. Signs and symptoms of osteosarcomas are worsening pain particularly at night, a mass that is tender and palpable, and patients may have fatigue, lethargy, malaise, fever, and pathological fracture. Diagnosis is confirmed through biopsy. Management includes surgical resection, chemotherapy, and radiation therapy (Pullan & Lotfollahzadeh, 2024).

Respiratory Illness

The most common types of respiratory illnesses seen in hospitalized school-aged children include pneumonia, influenza, and asthma. For discussion and management of these disorders, refer to the sections on toddlers and preschoolers.

Seizures and Epilepsy

Seizures and epilepsy can occur throughout childhood, including during the school age. Refer to the section on toddlers for discussion of these conditions and management.

Appendicitis

Acute appendicitis accounts for the most common cause of pediatric abdominal surgery. Symptoms generally escalate quickly and patients generally present emergently. The common reasons for acute appendicitis are bacterial infection, fecaliths, or tumors (Lotfollahzadeh et al., 2024). Symptoms of appendicitis may start as diffuse abdominal pain which then becomes localized to the right lower quadrant, anorexia, nausea, vomiting, diarrhea, malaise, and urinary urgency. Diagnosis includes CBC, C-reactive protein, and imaging such as ultrasound, CT, or MRI. Management of acute appendicitis includes surgical removal and antibiotics (Lotfollahzadeh et al., 2024).

Infections and Sepsis

School-aged children also may present with skin and soft tissue infections that result in hospitalizations, such as cellulitis, abscesses, bullous impetigo, and dermatitis with superinfection. For further descriptions and management of these conditions, refer to the section on toddlers above.

Pediatric sepsis varies from neonatal sepsis in risk factors and presentation. It may be difficult to determine the cause of sepsis, and literature states up to 75% of an unknown etiology of sepsis (Miranda & Nadel, 2023). Bacterial pathogens are the most common cause, followed by viral. Sepsis is defined as meeting the criteria for systemic inflammatory response syndrome (SIRS) and an infection that is suspected or confirmed. SIRS is defined as having two of the criteria or pyrexia (temperature greater than 38.5 °C) or hypothermia (temperature less than 36 °C), tachycardia or bradycardia, tachypnea or bradypnea, and abnormal white blood cell count or greater than 10% immature neutrophils (Miranda & Nadel, 2023). Immediate management of pediatric sepsis is needed to reduce associated morbidity and mortality. Interventions include antibiotics within one hour of recognizing sepsis, beginning with broad-spectrum antibiotics and then focusing on the causative organism. Fluid administration, vasoactive medications, corticosteroids, hemodynamic monitoring, nutrition, and ventilatory support may also be required (Miranda & Nadel, 2023).

Adolescents

The age of adolescents is considered 12 to 18 years old. Adolescents experience rapid and dramatic physical changes, including increases in height and development of primary and secondary sexual characteristics. Adolescents have increased nutritional requirements for calories, protein, calcium, iodine, iron, and B-complex vitamins. Cognitive abilities of adolescents are fully developed, such as logical and abstract thought, and deductive and analytical reasoning. Adolescents can form independent decisions, consider various options with problem-solving, and comprehend hypothetical situations (Maryniak, 2019).

Erikson's stage of development for adolescents is identity formation versus role confusion. Adolescents who attain identity formation show a solid belief of self and attentiveness to their duties, obligations, and trustworthiness. Adolescents who display role confusion have a poor sense of self and inadequate perception of their sexuality (Balasundaram & Avulakunta, 2023).

Adolescents may need reassurance that physical changes are normal and do not occur at the same time for each person. Privacy is essential for adolescents. Adolescents should be screened for nutritional and eating disorders, substance abuse, depression, and suicidal ideation. The independence and autonomy of adolescents can be respected by treating them as an adult, speaking directly to them, and encouraging self-care and decision-making. Acceptance of the adolescent should be demonstrated, while anticipating possible resistance and rebellion. Hospitalization may jeopardize the patient's evolving self-identity, including concern about separation from peers. The patient should be reassured, peer contact encouraged, and allowed to ask questions and articulation of fears.

Teaching includes the adolescent; and parents or caregivers should be included, but may require separate teaching. Nurses should respect the cognitive abilities of adolescents and explain all medical procedures. It is important to guide the adolescent toward healthy choices and discuss safety issues, which may be related to poor choices from peer pressure, such as substance use and abuse and sexuality. Specific information about sexuality should include correction of any misinformation from peers, discuss and encourage sexual responsibility, and teach about sexually transmitted diseases and pregnancy. Other important topics include depression and suicide, including encouragement of the use of stress-reduction techniques and discuss resources (Maryniak, 2019).

Behavioral Disorders

Behavioral illness and disorders can be seen in children and adolescents. Although behavioral changes such as rebellious or disrespectful behavior can be seen in adolescence, actual behavioral disorders can also occur. Behavioral disorders may be a comorbidity of a patient admitted for another reason.

Conduct disorder is defined as a behavioral pattern that disregards social norms and violates others' rights. It includes aggression to people or animals, destruction of property, deceitfulness, theft, and serious violations of rules (Mohan et al., 2023). Conduct disorder is seen in up to 10% of children and adolescents, with almost a four times greater incidence in males. Environmental factors including dysfunctional family dynamics, exposure to violence, and substance abuse exposure can contribute to the development of conduct disorder. Biology may also play a role, particularly testosterone levels, low dopamine, and potentially electrical brain activity. Conduct disorder that occurs earlier in childhood is associated with poor prognosis (Mohan et al., 2023). Management includes a combination of behavioral therapy for the patient and family, use of mood stabilizers, and management of any other comorbidities (Mohan et al., 2023).

Attention deficit hyperactivity disorder (ADHD) is a common behavioral disorder found in children and adolescents, affecting up to 10% of adolescents, with males at higher risk (Magnus et al., 2023; U.S. Department of Health & Human Services, 2025). Studies have shown structural changes in the brain and reduced activity in the frontostriatal region. Symptoms of ADHD include varying degrees of inattention, hyperactivity, and impulsivity (Magnus et al., 2023). Management of ADHD may include use of stimulants, non-stimulants including antidepressants or alpha agonists, and psychotherapy (Magnus et al., 2023).

Anxiety, Depression, and Suicidal Ideation

Anxiety disorders have been found to be increasing since the 2000 COVID pandemic, and up to 32% teenagers are affected (U.S. Department of Health & Human Services, 2025). Generalized anxiety disorder is the most common form, with risk factors including family history, physical illness and comorbidities, stress, substance use, and environmental factors (Munir & Takov, 2022). Symptoms of generalized anxiety disorder include excessive worry and anxiety for at least six months, difficulty controlling worry, anxiety associated with at least three other symptoms, and the anxiety resulting in significant distress. Management includes a combination of behavioral therapy and pharmacological treatment such as antidepressants, antipsychotics, or antianxiety medications (Munir & Takov, 2022).

Major depressive disorder has an average lifetime incidence of 12% and has been seen in childhood and adolescence, with females showing a higher incidence. Depression has a multifactorial cause including an imbalance in neurotransmitters, genetic predisposition, environmental factors such as substance abuse, and other psychosocial factors (Bains & Abdijadid, 2023). Symptoms include persistent feelings of sadness, loss of interest, hopelessness, irritability, changes in sleep, lack of energy, changes in appetite, and changes in concentration. Use of a validated depression tool is needed for diagnosis. Common management of depression includes behavioral therapy and antidepressants (Bains & Abdijadid, 2023).

Suicide has been identified as one of the leading causes of death between ages 10 and 24 and is associated with behavioral disorders and mental illness, including depression (Harmer et al., 2024). Physical illness, particularly chronic illness, also increases the risk of suicide, as well as patients who are male, members of the LGBTQ+ community, substance use, exposure to violence, and family or personal history of attempts. Suicidal ideation is thinking about ending one's life and may or may not include actual plans. It is important to use a validated tool to assess suicidal ideation and risk for suicide (Harmer et al., 2024).

Trauma

Trauma is another cause of admissions for children and adolescents and is the leading cause of death. Severity of trauma can vary and may include external damage, such as fractures and lacerations, and internal damage. Traumatic brain injury and hemorrhage are the most common reasons for morbidity and mortality (Theodorou et al., 2021). Deaths as a result of trauma peak immediately after the injury, minutes to hours after the event, and days to weeks after the injury as a result of organ failure or infection (Lee & Farrell, 2023). Full physical assessment is essential to determine injury and new or worsening symptoms. Frequent vital signs, neurological assessments, fluid management, and lab monitoring are also essential.

Seizures and Epilepsy

Seizures and epilepsy can occur throughout childhood, including during adolescence. Refer to the section on toddlers for discussion of these conditions and management.

Cancer

Although various forms of cancer can affect adolescents, Ewing sarcoma is one of the most common, being the second most common form of malignant bone cancer (Durer et al., 2024). There are no established risk factors for developing Ewing sarcoma, although it is more common in male patients and Caucasian ethnicity. Ewing sarcoma is usually found in the shaft of long bones but may appear in other locations. Pain (especially worsening at night), stiffness, and swelling over weeks to months are often primary symptoms. Fever and weight loss may be present with metastatic disease (Durer et al., 2024). Imaging such as x-rays, CT scans, and MRI along with biopsy can assist with staging. Chemotherapy, as well as surgery and radiation therapy, are primary management strategies. Ewing sarcoma that is not metastatic has a survival rate of 75–80% but drops to 30% with metastatic disease (Durer et al., 2024).

Appendicitis

Appendicitis is another reason that adolescents are admitted to hospital. For further discussion on appendicitis refer to the school-aged children section above.

Diabetes

Adolescents can also be admitted to hospital with type 1 or type 2 diabetes, DKA, or HHS. These can be a primary diagnosis or comorbidity. For further discussion and management, refer to the preschoolers' section on diabetes.

References

Adeyinka, A., & Kondamudi, N. P. (2023). *Hyperosmolar hyperglycemic syndrome*. StatPearls Publishing. https://www.ncbi.nlm.nih.gov/books/NBK482142/

American Cancer Society. (2025). *What is childhood leukemia?*. https://www.cancer.org/cancer/types/leukemia-in-children/about/what-is-childhood-leukemia.html

Bains, N., & Abdijadid, S. (2023). *Major depressive disorder*. StatPearls Publishing. https://www.ncbi.nlm.nih.gov/books/NBK559078/

Balasundaram, P., & Avulakunta, I. D. (2023). *Human growth and development*. StatPearls Publishing. https://www.ncbi.nlm.nih.gov/books/NBK567767/

Boktor, S. W., & Hafner, J. W. (2023). *Influenza*. StatPearls Publishing. https://www.ncbi.nlm.nih.gov/books/NBK459363/

Brigadoi, G., Rossin, S., Chiusaroli, L., Demarin, G. C., Maestri, L., Tesser, F., Matarazzo, M., Liberati, C., Barbieri, E., Giaquinto, C., Da Dalt, L., Bressan, S., & Donà, D. (2024). Impact of antibiotic stewardship on treatment of hospitalized children with skin and soft-tissue infections. *Children, 11*(11), 1325.

Carolan, P. (2023). *Pediatric bronchitis*. https://emedicine.medscape.com/article/1001332-overview

Damodharan, S., & Puccetti, D. (2023). Pediatric central nervous system tumor overview and emerging treatment considerations. *Brain Science, 13*(7), 1106.

Durer, S., Gasalberti, D. P., & Shaikh, H. (2024). *Ewing sarcoma*. StatPearls Publishing. https://www.ncbi.nlm.nih.gov/books/NBK559183/

Ebeledike, C., & Ahmad, T. (2023). *Pediatric pneumonia*. StatPearls Publishing. https://www.ncbi.nlm.nih.gov/books/NBK536940/

El-Mohandes, N., Yee, G., Bhutta, B. S., & Huecker, H. (2023). *Pediatric diabetic ketoacidosis*. StatPearls Publishing. https://www.ncbi.nlm.nih.gov/books/NBK470282/

Freedman, J., Leibovitzb, E., Sergienkoa, R., & Levya, A. (2024). Risk factors for hospitalization at the pediatric intensive care unit among infants and children younger than 5 years of age diagnosed with infectious diseases. *Pediatrics & Neonatology, 64*(2), 133–139.

Gardner, S. L., Carter, B. S., Enzman-Hines, M., & Niermeyer, S. (2020). *Merenstein & Gardner's handbook of neonatal intensive care* (9th ed.). Mosby Elsevier.

Harmer, B., Lee, S., Rizvi, A., & Saadabadi, A. (2024). *Suicidal ideation*. StatPearls Publishing. https://www.ncbi.nlm.nih.gov/books/NBK565877/

Herchline, T. (2024). *Cellulitis*. https://emedicine.medscape.com/article/214222-overview?_gl=1*1u2b2rz*_gcl_au*OTk3MDY2MTM0LjE3MzU3NjUwODY

Jain, H., Schweitzer, J. W., & Justice, N. A. (2023). *Respiratory syncytial virus infection in children*. StatPearls Publishing. https://www.ncbi.nlm.nih.gov/books/NBK459215/

Justice, N. A., Le, J. K., & Doerr, C. (2023). *Bronchiolitis (nursing)*. StatPearls Publishing. https://www.ncbi.nlm.nih.gov/sites/books/NBK568705/

Kemper, A. R., Newman, T. B., Slaughter, J. L., Maisels, M. J., Watchko, J. F., Downs, S. M., Grout, R. W., Bundy, D. G., Stark, A. R., Bogen, D. L., Holmes, A. V., Feldman-Winter, L. B., Bhutani, V. K., Brown, S. R., Maradiaga Panayotti, G. M., Okechukwu, K., Rappo, P. D., & Russell, T. L. (2022). Clinical practice guideline revision: Management of hyperbilirubinemia in the newborn infant 35 or more weeks of gestation. *Pediatrics, 150*(3), e2022058859.

Lee, L., & Farrell, C. (2023). Trauma management: Approach to the unstable child. *UpToDate.* https://www.uptodate.com/contents/trauma-management-approach-to-the-unstable-child

Leslie, S. W., Sajjad, H., & Murphy, P. B. (2023). *Wilms tumor*. StatPearls Publishing. https://www.ncbi.nlm.nih.gov/books/NBK442004/

Lizzo, J. M., Goldin, J., & Cortes, S. (2024). *Pediatric asthma*. StatPearls Publishing. https://www.ncbi.nlm.nih.gov/books/NBK551631/

Lotfollahzadeh, S., Lopez, R. A., & Deppen, J. G. (2024). *Appendicitis*. StatPearls Publishing. https://www.ncbi.nlm.nih.gov/books/NBK493193/

Lupo, P. J., & Spector, L. G. (2020). Cancer progress and priorities: Childhood cancer. *Cancer Epidemiol Biomarkers Preview, 29*(6), 1081–1094.

Magnus, W., Anilkumar, A. C., & Shaban, K. (2023). *Attention deficit hyperactivity disorder*. StatPearls Publishing. https://www.ncbi.nlm.nih.gov/books/NBK441838/

Mahapatra, S., & Challagundla, K. B. (2023). *Neuroblastoma*. StatPearls Publishing. https://www.ncbi.nlm.nih.gov/books/NBK448111/

Maryniak, K. (2019). *Professional nursing practice in the United States: An overview for international nurses, and those along the continuum from new graduates to experienced nurses*. Author.

Maryniak, K. (2023). *Controlling and preventing errors and pitfalls in neonatal care delivery*. Springer.

Minardi, C., Minacapelli, R., Valastro, P., Vasile, F., Pitino, S., Pavone, P., Astuto, M., & Murabito, P. (2019). Epilepsy in children: From diagnosis to treatment with focus on emergency. *Journal of Clinical Medicine, 8*(1), 39.

Miranda, M., & Nadel, S. (2023). Pediatric sepsis: A summary of current definitions and management recommendations. *Current Pediatric Report, 11*(2), 29–39.

Mohan, L., Yilanli, M., & Ray, S. (2023). *Conduct disorder*. StatPearls Publishing. https://www.ncbi.nlm.nih.gov/books/NBK470238/

Moon, A. (2023). *Impetigo*. https://emedicine.medscape.com/article/965254-overview#a4

Munir, S., & Takov, V. (2022). *Generalized anxiety disorder*. StatPearls Publishing. https://www.ncbi.nlm.nih.gov/books/NBK441870/

Panetti, B., Bucci, I., Di Ludovico, A., Pellegrino, G. M., Di Filippo, P., Di Pillo, S., Chiarelli, F., Attanasi, M., & Sferrazza Papa, G. F. (2024). Acute respiratory failure in children: A clinical update on diagnosis. *Children, 11*(10), 1232.

Prescilla, R. P. (2023). *Pediatric gastroenteritis*. Medscape. https://emedicine.medscape.com/article/964131-overview

Puckett, Y., & Chan, O. (2023). *Acute lymphocytic leukemia*. StatPearls Publishing. https://www.ncbi.nlm.nih.gov/books/NBK459149/

Pullan, J. E., & Lotfollahzadeh, S. (2024). *Primary bone cancer*. StatPearls Publishing. https://www.ncbi.nlm.nih.gov/books/NBK560830/

Rivera-Dominguez, G., & Ward, R. (2023). *Pediatric gastroenteritis*. StatPearls Publishing. https://www.ncbi.nlm.nih.gov/books/NBK499939/

Sapra, A., & Bhandari, P. (2023). *Diabetes*. StatPearls Publishing. https://www.ncbi.nlm.nih.gov/books/NBK551501

Singh, M., Alsaleem, M., & Gray, C. P. (2022). *Neonatal sepsis. StatPearls Publishing*. https://www.ncbi.nlm.nih.gov/books/NBK531478/

Sizar, O., & Carr, B. (2023). *Croup*. StatPearls Publishing. https://www.ncbi.nlm.nih.gov/books/NBK431070/

Springer, S. (2022). *Pediatric respiratory failure*. Medscape. https://emedicine.medscape.com/article/908172-overview?form=fpf

Theodorou, C. M., Galganski, L. A., Jurkovich, G. J., Farmer, D. L., Hirose, S., Stephenson, J. T., & Trappey, A. F. (2021). Causes of early mortality in pediatric trauma patients. *Journal of Trauma Acute Care Surgery, 90*(3), 574–581.

Thomas, M., & Bomar, P. A. (2023). *Upper respiratory tract infection*. StatPearls Publishing. https://www.ncbi.nlm.nih.gov/books/NBK532961/

U.S. Department of Health & Human Services. (2025). *Mental health for adolescents*. https://opa.hhs.gov/adolescent-health/mental-health-adolescents

Vakiti, A., Reynolds, S. B., & Mewawalla, P. (2024). *Acute myeloid leukemia*. StatPearls Publishing. https://www.ncbi.nlm.nih.gov/books/NBK507875/

Zieg, J., Ghose, S., & Raina, R. (2024). Electrolyte disorders related emergencies in children. *BMC Nephrology, 25*, 282.

Zohreh Jalali, S., Mahdipour, S., Asgarzad, R., & Saadat, F. (2024). Effect of intravenous immunoglobulin on the management of Rh- and ABO-mediated hemolytic disease of the newborn, *hematology, transfusion and cell. Therapy, 46*(supp. 5), S57–S64. ISSN 2531-1379. https://doi.org/10.1016/j.htct.2024.03.002

Predisposing and Contributing Factors for Nursing Errors

There are numerous factors that are involved with nursing errors and why they can occur. Errors should be viewed in terms of a "just culture," where the focus is on improving patient safety rather than blame. Just culture looks at accountability and faults within systems, rather than pointing fingers to blame one individual. When errors occur, processes often need improving or there is a lack of education. Just culture does not mean it is a blame-free environment, and if there is individual responsibility, then that person must have accountability (Marx, 2001; Maryniak, 2019).

By using the just culture framework, incidents are reviewed based on duties rather than the outcome. Individual duties include a duty to produce an outcome, a duty to follow a procedural rule, and a duty to avoid unjustifiable risk. For a duty to produce an outcome, there are no specific procedures or steps on how to do something, but as an individual, it is expected that you will have a defined result. There may be an acceptable rate of failure for expectations. With a duty to follow a procedural rule, the expectation is that as an individual we are expected to follow a procedure or policy in a specific way. The duty to avoid unjustifiable risk is described as an overarching duty for everyone. As individuals, generally we don't do anything that is intentionally reckless, however there are times when we may need to make a choice to do the right thing, but may breach and harm another value in the process; this is considered justifiable (van Baarle et al., 2022; Kim & Yu, 2021; Marx, 2001; Maryniak, 2019).

A breach of duty may occur from a variety of reasons, such as human error, at-risk behavior, and reckless behavior. Human error is an inadvertent action, a slip, lapse, or mistake. In these circumstances a genuine mistake is made. A human error may include a skill-based mistake, an omission or forgetfulness, or a knowledge-based error (Marx, 2001; Maryniak, 2019). An example of a human error is a nurse who is drawing up a medication in the medication room and is interrupted. When she asks her coworker to verify the dose, it is pointed out that she has drawn up the incorrect amount.

At-risk behavior is when someone chooses to do something that can inadvertently increase a chance for harm to occur. There is the potential for harm but it is not recognized by the person who is drifting away from consciously safer choices. The individual is aware that behavior is not following set practices, such as creating a workaround for a process. Many times, at-risk behaviors begin with system problems, such as ineffective processes, delays, or equipment problems. A workaround is found to deal with the system issue, but it creates a behavior that becomes dangerous (Marx, 2001; Maryniak, 2019). One example of this is that there are not enough barcode scanners on a particular unit. As a workaround, to ensure medications are given on time, nurses begin to override the barcode scanning rather than waiting to use the scanner. This is a system problem (not enough barcode scanners), but the nurses have found a workaround which is an at-risk behavior.

With reckless behavior, an individual actually chooses an action that knowingly puts themselves or others in harm's way. The risk is identified but ignored. The individual is aware that their behavior is reckless, and there is a conscious disregard of others (Marx, 2001; Maryniak, 2019). One example is narcotic diversion. The nurse is aware that it is illegal but does not stop the behavior.

Repetitive errors with patient safety also need to be addressed. Even if it is a human error each time, repetitiveness indicates a deeper problem (Marx, 2001; Maryniak, 2019). An example is a nurse who has repeated medication errors. The root is determined to be human error with each event, yet there are still multiple occasions of the issue, which increases patient risk.

When looking at how nursing errors occur, it is important to understand which contributing factors are involved. Contributing factors are those that can cause an error or determine the level of risk, directly or indirectly. An error may be a result from one or a combination of contributing factors, which may be related to human, environmental, or organizational considerations.

Multiple studies have determined that human errors such as slips and lapses are the most common cause of nursing errors. Personal and environmental factors are frequently contributing causes for human errors. One condition that can lead to slips and lapses involves personal health status. This includes fatigue, sleep deprivation, and illness. Other physical signs, such as those indicating burnout, have been noted in studies which can be related to long hours and lack of breaks. Stress at work, lack of assertiveness, and personality also contributed to personal health. A busy work environment, distractions, interruptions, pressure from others, or time limitations can also increase the likelihood of human errors. Staff skill mix and workload is commonly identified as contributing to errors. This includes the volume of admissions, discharges, and transfers. Staffing with heavy patient loads and multitasking were other factors where omissions and violations occurred more often. Patient acuity was another condition identified as a contributing factor. This was particularly true when combined with other factors, often shown in medication errors of wrong time or dose omission. Studies have also demonstrated that short staffing is also a factor for errors, particularly when added to skill mix of staff, workload, and patient acuity (Donaldson et al., 2021; Sameera et al., 2021).

Examples of slips and lapses involving medications include misidentifying either a medication or patient. Contributing causes are misreading labels or documentation, look-alike, soundalike medications or patient names, lack of concentration, complacency, and carelessness. Further descriptions of errors will be covered in Chap. 3.

Knowledge-based mistakes were also noted in studies, but were less frequent. This included lack of knowledge about disease processes, understanding about medications being administered or equipment that was being used, as well as unfamiliarity with the patient. Lack of critical thinking may be related to knowledge, personal, or environmental factors (Donaldson et al., 2021; Sameera et al., 2021).

Written communication in studies included illegible and unclear documentation. Transcription errors also contributed to medication and procedure errors. These types of contributing factors were associated with facilities who still use written documentation or during downtime procedures. Other sources of inadequate written communication were a lack of appropriate policies, procedures, or protocols. Verbal communications, such as handoffs or interdisciplinary communications, were also noted in studies as contributing to errors (Badgery-Parker et al., 2024; Sameera et al., 2021).

Supplies and storage are also associated with errors. Logistics related to a unit or ward stock contributed to errors with medication and procedure times or omission, including medication or supply misplacement. Delays in delivery of medication or treatment, or unavailable medications and supplies were also sources of errors. Difficulties with equipment is another contributing condition for errors. Malfunctioning equipment, unfamiliarity with or unclear equipment design, and insufficient availability of equipment contributed to errors (Badgery-Parker et al., 2024; Donaldson et al., 2021).

Deliberate violations were not commonly seen in studies, and one cannot infer that there was malicious or ill intent. In these studies, violations were occurrences in which the nurses knew that processes were not followed, were situational, and were related to trusting colleagues, lack of appropriate protocols, patient acuity, and staff. The violations noted in studies related to medication errors were intentionally giving medications early or late, and administering medication without a signed order (Badgery-Parker et al., 2024).

Reckless behaviors that lead to errors can include use of controlled substances at work, deliberately tampering with equipment or medications, or knowingly practicing outside of the scope of practice. These types of behaviors are not typical, but are dealt with through corrective action (van Baarle et al., 2022).

References

Badgery-Parker, T., Li, L., Fitzpatrick, E., Mumford, V., Raban, M. Z., & Westbrook, J. K. (2024). Child age and risk of medication error: A multisite children's hospital study. *The Journal of Pediatrics, 272*, 114087.

Donaldson, L., Ricciardi, W., Sheridan, S., & Tartaglia, R. (Eds.). (2021). *Textbook of patient safety and clinical risk management*. Springer.

Kim, B. B., & Yu, S. (2021). Effects of just culture and empowerment on patient safety activities of hospital nurses. *Healthcare, 9*(10), 1324.

Marx, D. (2001). *Patient safety and the just culture: A primer for health care executives*. Trustees of Columbia University.

Maryniak, K. (2019). *Professional nursing practice in the United States: An overview for international nurses, and those along the continuum from new graduates to experienced nurses*. Author.

Sameera, V., Bindra, A., & Rath, G. P. (2021). Human errors and their prevention in healthcare. *Journal of Anaesthesiology and Clinical Pharmacology, 37*(3), 328–335.

van Baarle, E., Hartman, L., Rooijakkers, S., Wallenburg, I., Weenink, J. W., Bal, R., & Widdershoven, G. (2022). Fostering a just culture in healthcare organizations: Experiences in practice. *BMC Health Services Research, 22*, 1035.

Types of Errors

Approximately 9.5% of all patient deaths annually in the United States are caused from medical errors (Institute of Medicine, 2000; Johns Hopkins Medicine, 2016), and that includes pediatric patients. It is difficult to quantify the statistics of medical errors with these vulnerable patients, but errors can include medication errors, delayed care, hospital acquired infections, errors with equipment or devices, errors with procedures, and accidents, to name a few (ElMeneza et al., 2020). Nurses play a key role in the prevention of errors, and unfortunately, they also play a key role in making errors. Many errors are due to poor processes or failure to follow policies and procedures.

Medical errors can be tragic in pediatric settings and rarely does a single problem or issue lead to an error. Good systems should have stable layers of defense against errors, but factors such as deviations from processes can cause a "Swiss cheese" effect which in turn leads to an error. System layers are at the point of patient care, individual healthcare professionals, the healthcare team, and the organization itself. Active failures in the system, latent conditions, human factors, and environmental hazards contribute to errors (Agency for Healthcare Research and Quality [AHRQ], 2019).

There are multiple common events that occur with children and these unfortunate events can result in temporary or permanent harm, including death. Some common events are hospital acquired infections, adverse drug events, intravenous catheter extravasation, accidental extubation, and intracranial hemorrhage and ischemia. Other events include misidentification errors for medications, diagnostic tests, treatment, and documentation (Gardner et al., 2020; Verklan et al., 2021).

Errors Associated with Hospital-Acquired Conditions

Although not all patient harm is associated with errors, some errors can result in hospital-acquired conditions. Nurses commonly perform what's referred to as "stacking," when there are multiple cognitive processes and competing priorities in the mind. The ability to manage many plans and thoughts for carrying out patient care through stacking can be impeded by the environment, changing situations, interruptions, delays, or time constraints. The practice environment consists of work design, adequate staffing, appropriate skill mix and assignments, organizational management, policies, resources, and the culture of the work environment (Al-ghraiybah, et al., 2021).

Hospital-acquired conditions (HACs) for the pediatric patient include central line–associated bloodstream infections (CLABSIs), catheter-associated urinary tract infections (CAUTIs), ventilator-associated pneumonia (VAP), and hospital-acquired infections (also referred to as nosocomial infections). Healthcare associated infections are also known as hospital acquired infections or nosocomial infections. These infections are transmitted to the child in the environment, and may be caused from improper hand hygiene, invasive tubes and lines, peripheral lines, central lines, catheters, and ventilators. A CLABSI is a healthcare associated infection, and risk factors are an increased risk with extended dwell time, improper sterile technique with insertion, dressing changes, poor hand hygiene, and open lines. The risk of CAUTI is also higher the longer the catheter is in place, with improper technique for insertion, catheter maintenance, and perineal care. CAUTIs can cause bacteremia, meningitis, cystitis, and osteomyelitis. VAP is a healthcare associated infection where the pneumonia may be caused by gram-positive or gram-negative bacteria. Risk factors for VAP include prematurity, low birthweight, duration of ventilation, use of opiates, reintubation, frequent suctioning, enteral feeds, parenteral nutrition, steroids, poor oral care, and transfusion (Gardner et al., 2020; Kenner et al., 2019)

Errors that can contribute to hospital-acquired conditions include lack of appropriate or timely assessment. Assessment can be interrupted, delayed, or missed, due to the practice environment or issues affecting cognitive stacking (Al-ghraiybah et al., 2021; Sameera et al., 2021). Skin assessments are required frequently. Patients on ventilators should be assessed at least daily for continuation. Assessment of lines and drains are also necessary on a consistent basis. Missed assessments can lead to increased risk for CLABSIs and UTIs. Delayed or missing assessments of peripheral intravenous (IV) sites may also lead to infiltration or extravasation.

Delays, missed care opportunities, or not performing interventions can also occur, which are errors that can predispose patients to hospital-acquired conditions or falls (Al-ghraiybah et al., 2021; Sameera et al., 2021). Examples can be lack of perineal care or cleansing for patients with urinary catheter usage, which can lead to UTIs. Inappropriate cleaning of central line access can create increased risk of CLABSIs. Failure to provide appropriate oral care can contribute to development of ventilator-associated pneumonia (VAP).

Failures in communication, both written and verbal, can also create errors (Sameera et al., 2021). Verbal communication mainly occurs with report and handoffs. Using checklists and standardized tools to provide verbal communication can create more complete reports and ensure that vital patient information is passed along. Examples of communication tools may be SBAR or I-PASS (Miller, 2021; Sameera et al., 2021) (see also Chap.6). Additionally, providing a bedside report with the offgoing nurse, the oncoming nurse, and the family (if able) can ensure that there is a verbal and visual handoff, which can increase patient safety (Bigani & Correia, 2018).

Complete documentation of assessment, interventions, and nursing care planning is essential. Assessments should be done real time, and documentation of lines and drains must be clear as well (Maryniak, 2021). Even with complete documentation, nurses caring for patients must read what is charted and apply it. An important consideration to assist with critical thinking is looking for trends in patient care status. Identifying and applying trends is helpful in proactively planning and intervening on behalf of the patient (Maryniak, 2021).

Errors Associated with Developmental Stages

Children, as vulnerable patients, have additional considerations for the developmental stages they are at. Infants are completely reliant on others for their care. They cannot verbally communicate, and nonverbal cues must be interpreted to determine their needs such as pain or hunger. They are unable to comply with simple commands, although there is limited ability as they near toddlerhood (Maryniak, 2019). Safety considerations include ensuring they have rails up on cribs or doors closed on incubators. Infants also frequently put objects in their mouth, so objects and equipment must not be available within their reach.

Toddlers are at high risk for falls and injury due to their high energy and activity. As previously discussed, there is a rapid development of motor skills during this time period, but coordination is still poor (Maryniak, 2019). Toddlers still have limited verbal skills and there is an emphasis on nonverbal communication. They can begin to participate in care but may be impulsive or noncooperative. The inability to recognize danger can increase risks of injury such as falls, choking, and poisoning.

As described earlier, advancing development of children includes ability to understand and communicate. Preschoolers need correct information provided to them, including if procedures will hurt. However, there may not be cooperation, and involvement of others such as caregivers is necessary for safety. Distractions, demonstrations, and offering choices can also be good strategies. Preschoolers still cannot comprehend danger and need rules and boundaries as well as supervision. Falls can occur as a result of poor judgement. Exploring behaviors in the preschooler can also increase safety risks related to objects, equipment, and medication.

School-aged children can participate more in making decisions with guidance and should be encouraged to care for themselves when appropriate. It is important to provide correct information and allow school-aged children to ask questions and examine equipment. If school-aged children hurt themselves, such as a fall, they may be embarrassed to let someone know.

Adolescents have an increased level of independence and decision-making. Correct information should be provided and guidance is required to make appropriate and safe decisions. Some adolescents may have noncompliance related to their still-developing thought processes. Fear and anxiety are common and should be communicated, with reassurance provided.

Pain in the child can create physiological and behavioral outcomes, and is not easily identified. The sympathetic nervous system of the child can have a decreased response with persistent and painful stimuli, which may obscure signs of pain or discomfort. General pain contributes to hypoxia, hypercarbia, acidosis, hyperglycemia, and respiratory distress. Pain related to invasive procedures contribute to increased hypoxemic events and alterations in oxygenation (Motluk, 2019). Strategies for providing developmentally appropriate care and pain management are essential with pediatric care.

Errors Associated with Medical Devices and Equipment

The use of equipment and medical devices is essential in caring for ill children. Research studies show that intravenous infusion pumps and respiratory equipment were most commonly associated with equipment errors. Some consequences of errors with equipment or medical devices include inadequate or inappropriate ventilation, pneumothorax, atelectasis, skin integrity issues and damage, catheter occlusion, disruption of thermoregulation, and prolonged length of stay (Brado et al., 2021; ELMeneza et al., 2020).

Equipment malfunction can cause errors which may have significant effects on the children. Malfunction can be from actual device failure, inadequate maintenance such as calibration, lack of technical support, equipment assembly issues, or poor equipment design. Lack of appropriate equipment is also associated with errors (Brado et al., 2021; ELMeneza et al., 2020).

Other causes of equipment or medical device errors is related to human factors. These include distraction, fatigue, inadequate training, lack of experience, poor or unavailable policies and procedures, miscommunications, and time constraints (Brado et al., 2021; ELMeneza et al., 2020).

Errors Associated with Identification

Children are at a higher risk for identification errors as hospital bands may not be placed due to the fragility of skin or that the patient or caregivers do not want them on. Placement of identification bands on pediatric patients is crucial to verify identifiers such as name and birthdate. Studies have examined errors with children, including sentinel events, in which identification of the patient was a key factor. Errors associated with misidentification include procedural, medications, administration of breastmilk or formula, and incorrect laboratory or radiology results (Wallace, 2016).

Errors Related to Procedures

There are multiple errors that can occur with procedures. The most common errors are mislabeled or unlabeled laboratory specimens, hemolyzed or insufficient blood samples, and wrong patient reports. Failure to perform procedures correctly are another type of error, which can be the result of lack of knowledge or experience, time constraints, inappropriate or absent procedural standards, and environmental effects. Incorrect procedures can include vascular procedures such as use of catheters, respiratory procedures, blood sampling, phototherapy, blood transfusion, and management of urinary catheters (Hjelmgren et al., 2022)

Errors Affecting Skin Integrity

Children are at high risk for damage to the skin related to the poor integumentary system, and there are higher risks with premature infants. Diligence is required to support skin integrity as a break in this first line of defense can easily create infection and sepsis in the child. Skin tears, epidermal stripping, and pressure injuries can occur. Skin injury from mechanical force is commonly seen with children, estimated at 40–45%. Medical devices contribute to skin injury such as vascular catheters, respiratory equipment, and use of adhesives. Infiltration and extravasation are also seen with pediatric patients (August et al., 2021).

Medication Errors

It is difficult to quantify how many medication errors occur as there is no centralized reporting system for all errors. It is theorized that children are three times more likely to be exposed to a medication error than adults (Marufu et al., 2022). Some studies show that medication errors can occur between 32%–94% of the time, with 38% of those errors attributed to nursing (Salar et al., 2020). Other studies specific to children demonstrated prescribing errors can be as high as 55%, and administration errors average 30% of the time (D'Errico et al., 2022). The most common medication errors by nursing are wrong dose, wrong time, omissions, and wrong medication (MacDowell et al., 2021).

Just as previously discussed, there are multiple contributing factors, which can lead to medication errors. Slips and lapses were identified in studies as a common cause of medication errors, such as miscalculations for weight-based drugs, while communications, supplies, and inadequate processes also contributed. Moreover, lack of education, personal factors (including noncompliance with safety practices), and poor system features (such a lack of effective bar-coded scanning systems) can create a high risk for medication errors (Maryniak, 2023).

Errors Related to Missed Nursing Care

Missed nursing care can lead to errors with children. Children can be cared for in a variety of settings, and there are many factors which can lead to missing nursing care opportunities. The most commonly found reasons cited in studies for missing nursing care are an emergency or deterioration of another patient. Studies discuss the most frequent areas of pediatric nursing care that are missed and include providing developmental care, giving emotional support to parents, ensuring all important information is given during report, performing hand hygiene at all five moments of opportunity, providing skin care, assessing and cleaning eyes of children under phototherapy, and repositioning (Gathara et al., 2020; Kim & Chae, 2022).

References

Agency for Healthcare Research and Quality (AHRQ). (2019). *Nurse bedside shift report: Implementation handbook.* https://www.ahrq.gov/sites/default/files/wysiwyg/professionals/systems/hospital/engagingfamilies/strategy3/Strat3_Implement_Hndbook_508.pdf

Al-ghraiybah, T., Sim, J., & Lago, L. (2021). The relationship between the nursing practice environment and five nursing-sensitive patient outcomes in acute care hospitals: A systematic review. *Nursing Open, 8*(5), 2262–2271.

August, D., Kandasamy, Y., Ray, R., Lindsay, D., & New, K. (2021). Fresh perspectives on hospital-acquired pediatric skin injury period prevalence from a multicenter study. *The Journal of Perinatal & Pediatric Nursing, 35*(3), 275–283.

Bigani, D. K., & Correia, A. M. (2018). On the same page: Nurse, patient, and family perceptions of change-of-shift bedside report. *Journal of Pediatric Nursing, 41*, 84–89.

References

Brado, L., Tippmann, S., Daniel, S., Jonas, J., Dorothea, P., et al. (2021). Patterns of safety incidents in a pediatric intensive care unit. *Frontiers in Pediatrics, 9*. https://www.frontiersin.org/articles/10.3389/fped.2021.664524/full

D'Errico, S., Zanon, M., Radaelli, D., Padovano, M., Santurro, A., Scopetti, M., Frati, P., & Fineschi, V. (2022). Medication errors in pediatrics: Proposals to improve the quality and safety of care through clinical risk management. *Frontiers in Medicine, 14*(8), 814100. https://doi.org/10.3389/fmed.2021.814100

ELMeneza, S., Elnaser, A., Elmoean, A., & Elmoneem, N. (2020). Study of medical errors triggered by medical devices in pediatric intensive care unit. *Edelweiss Pediatric Journal, 1*(1), 7–12.

Gardner, S. L., Carter, B. S., Enzman-Hines, M., & Niermeyer, S. (2020). *Merenstein & Gardner's handbook of neonatal intensive care* (9th ed.). Mosby Elsevier.

Gathara, D., Serem, G., Murphy, G., Obengo, A., Tallam, E., et al. (2020). Missed nursing care in newborn units: A cross-sectional direct observational study. *BMJ Quality & Safety, 29*, 19–30.

Hjelmgren, H., Ygge, B. M., Nordlund, B., & Nina Andersson, N. (2022). Nurses' experiences of blood sample collection from children: A qualitative study from Swedish paediatric hospital care. *BMC Nursing, 21*, 62. https://doi.org/10.1186/s12912-022-00840-2

Institute of Medicine. (2000). *To err is human: Building a safer health system*. National Academies Press.

Johns Hopkins Medicine. (2016). *Study suggests medical errors now third leading cause of death in the U.S.* https://www.hopkinsmedicine.org/news/media/releases

Kenner, C., Altimier, L., & Boykova, M. (Eds.). (2019). *Comprehensive pediatric nursing care* (6th ed.). Springer.

Kim, S., & Chae, S. (2022). Missed nursing care and its influencing factors among pediatric intensive care unit nurses: A descriptive study. *Child Health Nursing Research, 28*(2), 142–153.

MacDowell, P., Cabri, A., & Davis, M. (2021). Medication administration errors. *Patient Safety Network*. https://psnet.ahrq.gov/primer/medication-administration-errors

Marufu, T. C., Bower, R., Hendron, E., & Manning, J. C. (2022). Nursing interventions to reduce medication errors in paediatrics and neonates: Systematic review and meta-analysis. *Journal of Pediatric Nursing, 62*, E139–E147.

Maryniak, K. (2019). *Professional nursing practice in the United States: An overview for international nurses, and those along the continuum from new graduates to experienced nurses*. Author.

Maryniak, K. (2021). *Documentation for nurses* (4th ed. (ebook)). Elite Healthcare.

Maryniak, K. (2023). *Controlling and preventing errors and pitfalls in neonatal care delivery*. Springer.

Miller, D. (2021). I-PASS as a nursing communication tool. *Pediatric Nursing, 47*(1), 30–37.

Motluk, A. (2019). Poorly managed childhood pain can have lifelong consequences. *Canadian Medical Association Journal, 191*(27), E771–E772. https://doi.org/10.1503/cmaj.109-5768

Salar, A., Kiani, F., & Rezaee, N. (2020). Preventing the medication errors in hospitals: A qualitative study. *International Journal of Africa Nursing Sciences, 13, 100235.*

Sameera, V., Bindra, A., & Rath, G. P. (2021). Human errors and their prevention in healthcare. *Journal of Anaesthesiology and Clinical Pharmacology, 37*(3), 328–335.

Verklan, M., Walden, M., & Forest, S. (Eds.). (2021). *Core curriculum for neonatal intensive care* (6th ed.). Elsevier.

Wallace, S. (2016). Newborns pose unique identification challenges. *Pennsylvania Patient Safety Advisory, 13*(2), 42–50.

Consequences of Nursing Errors

4

Not all errors cause actual patient harm but there is a much higher risk for creating harm. Consequences related to errors have more detrimental effects with pediatric patients.

Levels of Harm

Nursing errors can be associated with a variety of patient outcomes. A near miss is when an error doesn't actually reach the patient, but has the potential to cause harm. A near miss is an opportunity to identify a breakdown in the process before patient harm actually occurs (American Society for Healthcare Risk Management, 2014; Maryniak, 2019). One example of a near miss is a nurse who examines syringe labeled for a dispensed single dose of intravenous metoclopramide. She sees that the syringe contains a solution that is cloudy. The nurse knows that IV metoclopramide should be clear. She does not give the medication, and reports the incident to pharmacy, returning the syringe that was dispensed.

No harm means that although an event reached a patient, there was no harm (American Society for Healthcare Risk Management, 2014; Maryniak, 2019). An illustration of an incident with no harm is an order for a pediatric patient is changed to increase oral feedings and decrease IV fluid rate. The nurse doesn't see the order at the time of the oral feeding and this change isn't made immediately. Rather, the change of the volume of oral feedings and decreased IV fluids is made three hours later. This is an error of delay, but there was no resulting harm to the patient.

Mild harm includes minimal symptoms or injury with minor interventions, observation, or increased length of stay (American Society for Healthcare Risk Management, 2014; Maryniak, 2019). An instance of mild harm is a new nurse who is still learning about handling pediatric patients with developmentally supportive strategies. He is preparing to weigh the infant patient on the warmer and lifts the child off the warmer to zero the scale. He does not contain the child, and when lifted the child demonstrates an abrupt startle reflex, with splaying and grimacing. The child is placed back on the warmer for the weight, and continues to show distressing behavior as well as desaturations, tachypnea, and tachycardia, followed by a brief episode of apnea and bradycardia. When the patient is repositioned and contained, vital signs return to baseline and the patient's behaviors become relaxed. Although there was initial harm, there was no lasting harm.

Moderate harm means that the patient has bodily or psychological injury which affects the quality of life or function (American Society for Healthcare Risk Management, 2014; Maryniak, 2019). An example is a nurse who does not perform blood sampling via a heel stick appropriately. She uses a lancet that is too big for the patient's size, and punctures deeply near the heel. Nurses assess the site, which becomes reddened, swollen, and painful to the patient. The patient develops osteomyelitis, confirmed by testing. Management includes antibiotics, wound care, and minimal handling. This is moderate harm as there was patient injury which affected the patient's quality of life and additional treatment which potentially increased length of stay. The child recovers from the infection without apparent long-term consequences.

Severe harm indicates physical or psychological injury to a patient, which significantly affects function or quality of life (American Society for Healthcare Risk Management, 2014; Maryniak, 2019). One case of severe harm is a patient who had extravasation from a peripheral infusion of TPN located in the right hand. The incident happened during a very busy shift and the nurse did not assess the IV site for several hours. When she checked the site, it was blistering and discolored, and the hand and arm were cold and severely swollen. She immediately removed the cannula, attempted aspiration, and gave hyaluronidase per provider's order. The hand and part of the arm became necrotic, and a plastic surgeon was consulted. It was determined that plastic surgery was warranted, and there was a high likelihood that future mobility of the hand and arm would be impacted. The harm was severe, with significant effects to the patient's quality of life.

Death is the last patient outcome as a result of an event (American Society for Healthcare Risk Management, 2014; Maryniak, 2019). Some well-known examples, unfortunately, are medication overdoses from either inadvertently mixing inappropriately, dispensing incorrectly or having wrong doses available, incorrect weight-based calculations, or administration of incorrect concentrations, leading to overdoses. As a result, multiple children died from these errors.

Avoidable Harm

Errors related to the care of children can not only harm the one patient, but can possibly harm others. Failure to perform hand hygiene or use PPE appropriately can increase the risk of exposure to the healthcare professional through contamination. This in turn can put the caregiver at risk, as well as increase the risk of spreading infectious diseases to other patients. A higher chance of contagion spread to other patients or even loved ones of the healthcare professional at home may occur (Fan et al., 2020). Examples include the spread of MDROs in a hospital setting, such as MRSA in a pediatric intensive care unit (NICU). MRSA can often be spread by individuals who are colonized with the bacteria, usually from a community-acquired setting. Many studies have shown that outbreaks in a pediatric setting can be traced to a healthcare professional who unknowingly passes along MRSA to these vulnerable patients (Brown et al., 2019). Diligent hand hygiene and appropriate use of PPE can help prevent these outbreaks, along with other strategies.

Avoidable patient harm that can occur from errors can also increase morbidity and mortality. Both short-term and long-term effects may be seen. Hospital-acquired conditions such as CLABSIs, CAUTIs, VAP, pressure injuries, falls, and other hospital-acquired infections can cause unnecessary patient pain and suffering, complex conditions, potential disability, and impact on both physical and psychological states. Other consequences include longer lengths of stay (and all of the associated risks with that), as well as increased costs to the healthcare system (Panagioti et al., 2019).

Long-Term Harmful Effects

Errors and harm for pediatric patients can increase long-term harmful effects to them physically, as well as have other chronic effects on the patients and families. Psychological, social, and emotional effects to patients and family members may last throughout their lives as a result of the trauma and loss of trust. There can also be financial consequences that occur from lasting physical harm (Ottosen et al., 2021).

Central Line–Associated Blood Stream Infections

A CLABSI is a central line–associated blood stream infection. The most vulnerable patients for developing CLABSIs include pediatric intensive care patients due to the high utilization rates of central lines. CLABSI rates for pediatric populations have been 1.1–2.5 cases per 1000 patient line days in the United States, including acute care and ambulatory settings (Hsu et al., 2020). Within pediatric populations, the highest rates are for patients in intensive care units and oncology patients. The risk for developing a CLABSI increases with the length of time the line is in place (Hsu et al., 2020). CLABSI is associated with high mortality and morbidity among the healthcare acquired infections, due to bacteremia or fungal invasion, at a rate of 20,000–30,000 people each year (Agency for Healthcare Research & Quality [AHRQ], 2020). Even in situations where there is no patient death, developing a CLABSI can cause the pediatric patient pain and stress.

Catheter-Associated Urinary Tract Infections

A CAUTI is a urinary tract infection that is related to the use of an indwelling urinary catheter. CAUTIs commonly occur with pediatric patients, and the average rate of CAUTI in pediatrics in 1.33 per 1000 patient line days (Hsu et al., 2020). Most pediatric CAUTIs are from E.coli as the invading pathogen. Like CLABSIs, the risk for developing a CAUTI increases with the length of time the line is in place (Hsu et al., 2020). Other risks for CAUTIs are prematurity, comorbidities, and impaired immunity. Developing a CAUTI can be painful and create other patient complications, including sepsis.

Ventilator-Associated Pneumonia

Ventilator-associated events (VAEs) are those that cause deterioration in respiratory status after a period of stability or improvement on the ventilator, with evidence of infection or inflammation, and laboratory evidence of respiratory infection. Ventilator-associated pneumonia (VAP) is one form of VAE and is a common hospital-acquired infection in intensive care units. VAP rates in pediatric ICUs range from 1 to 63 cases per 1000 ventilator days (Antalová et al., 2022). The length of time for intubation is a risk factor, and studies estimate up to 20% of critically ill children develop VAP after 48 hours of intubation (Wang et al., 2021). VAP is associated with long-term outcomes, including chronic lung disease as well as pediatric mortality, with mortality rates as high as 16% (Wang et al., 2021).

Disruption of Skin Integrity

Pressure injuries are those that cause localized injury to the skin and underlying tissue. These injuries may or may not be pressure ulcers, and are generally seen over a bony prominence. Pressure injuries are caused by pressure and shear, or the combination of both. Children are vulnerable due to fragile skin, lack of subcutaneous fat, limited mobility, disease processes, use of devices and adhesives, and incontinence. Studies of skin injury with pediatric patients estimate the prevalence as 12–20% (Gao et al., 2024). Pediatric skin injury significantly increases the risk of developing infections and sepsis.

Harm from Medication Errors

Medication errors can range in the degree of patient harm, from near misses to patient death. As previously discussed, the rates of medication errors occurring with pediatric populations is much higher than adult patients. Dosing errors are the most commonly reported medication errors with pediatric patients (Shawahna et al., 2022). In addition to incorrect dose, other recurrent medication errors with pediatric patients include dose omission, wrong route of administration, wrong intervals between medications, and medication administration after discontinuation by a provider (D'Errico et al., 2022; Eslami et al., 2019).

Medication errors may also cause adverse drug events (ADEs), which are often associated with patient harm. Errors associated with high-risk medications are those that often lead to severe harm, disability, or even death. Preventable patient injury from medication errors can have a long-term impact on the patient and family (Afreen et al., 2021).

An ADE is harm that occurs as a result of a medication. Not all ADEs are result of an error. For example, heparin induced thrombocytopenia (HIT) is a reaction that occurs from the use of heparin. HIT is considered an ADE, even when the medication is administered appropriately. A preventable ADE is one that is associated with a medication error which causes patient harm. It is estimated that about 5% of all hospitalized patients experience a preventable ADE (PSNet, 2019). Risk factors for an ADE in hospital are neonatal and pediatric patients, polypharmacy, high alert medications, use of look-alike, soundalike medications, and ineffective processes or noncompliance with safe medication administration (PSNet, 2019). Mortality for pediatric patients is estimated at 0.13% of those reported ADEs worldwide (Montastruc, 2023).

The Impact of Falls

Falls are defined as an unplanned descent to the floor. In the United States alone, approximately 700,000 to 1,000,000 patients fall in healthcare settings each year, with 250,000 suffering from injury (LeLaurin & Shorr, 2019). Injuries associated with falls may range from bruises, lacerations, and fractures to internal bleeding and death.

Widespread Effects of Patient Harm

Errors that occur in healthcare can also have effects on others. Trust between the family and the healthcare team can be negatively affected by an error. This can occur even if there is disclosure about the error, although the impact on the family's perception may be improved with disclosure. The Institute of Medicine's report, *To Err is Human* (2000), errors are systemic but often decrease trust in the healthcare professional who made the error. Institutions that are not proactive, transparent, or create action when an error occurs can cause a patient to feel betrayed. This betrayal is often directed at the healthcare professional, rather than at the organization that had systemic issues. Families who have pediatric patients, particularly those who are sick and critically ill, are in a state of crisis. They may be experiencing grief, fear, and life stress from the situation alone. Errors in the care of their baby can exacerbate these emotions even if there is no patient harm. And if errors cause pediatric harm or even death, these events are significantly intensified, with long-term effects on the family members as well as the patients.

The healthcare professional themselves may also be impacted by an error. Second victim syndrome is a term for the healthcare professional, such as a nurse, who has committed an error. The professional feels responsible, particularly if the error is associated with a poor outcome. The person may feel shame, guilt, anxiety, grief, depression, compassion dissatisfaction, burnout, secondary traumatic stress, and physical manifestations. The psychological effects are not just about responsibility, but goes deeper to where the healthcare professional can be traumatized as a result of the event (Ozeke et al., 2019).

Nursing errors can also impact the organization itself. Patient harm resulting from errors has financial effects. There are higher costs associated with longer lengths of stay. And hospital-acquired conditions are not reimbursed by insurance companies. The additional costs for a patient who develops a CLABSI is an average of $48,000 (U.S. dollars), and CAUTI adds approximately $31,000 (Sentiff et al., 2023). VAP has an average cost of $27,000 (Ladbrook et al., 2021). Pediatric sepsis has costs up to $129,000 per case, many of which are results of hospital acquired infection (Salman et al., 2020). Additional costs for ADEs are estimated at $3500, (Encinosa et al., 2023).

Additionally, there may be lawsuits against an organization for patient harm that is caused by error. The lawsuits themselves can cost an organization financially, but the public perception of the organization may also be affected. Long-term, the organization's reputation may be damaged, which can lead to further negative financial impact (Alabdaly et al., 2024).

References

Afreen, N., Padilla-Tolentino, E., & McGinnis, B. (2021). Identifying potential high-risk medication errors using telepharmacy and a web-based survey tool. *Innovations in Pharmacy, 12*(1), 10.

Agency for Healthcare Research and Quality (AHRQ). (2020). *Guide: Purpose and use of CLABSI tools*. https://www.ahrq.gov/hai/clabsi-tools/guide.html

Alabdaly, A., Hinchcliff, R., Debono, D., & Hor, S. (2024). Relationship between patient safety culture and patient experience in hospital settings:

A scoping review. *BMC Health Service Research, 24*, 906. https://doi.org/10.1186/s12913-024-11329-w

American Society for Healthcare Risk Management. (2014). *Serious safety events: A focus on harm classification: Deviation in care as link.* http://www.ashrm.org/pubs/files/white_papers/SSE-2_getting_to_zero-9-30-14.pdf.

Antalová, N., Klučka, J., Říhová, M., Poláčková, S., Pokorná, A., & Štourač, P. (2022). Ventilator-associated pneumonia prevention in pediatric patients: Narrative review. *Children, 9*(10), 1540. https://doi.org/10.3390/children9101540

Brown, N., Reacher, M., Rice, W., Roddick, I., Reeve, L., et al. (2019). An outbreak of methicillin-resistant staphylococcus aureus colonization in a pediatric intensive care unit: Use of a case-control study to investigate and control it and lessons learnt. *Journal of Hospital Infections, 103*(1), 35–43.

D'Errico, S., Zanon, M., Radaelli, D., Padovano, M., Santurro, A., Scopetti, M., Frati, P., & Fineschi, V. (2022). Medication errors in pediatrics: Proposals to improve the quality and safety of care through clinical risk management. *Frontiers in Medicine, 14*(8), 814100. https://doi.org/10.3389/fmed.2021.814100

Encinosa, W., Moon, K., Figueroa, J., & Elias, Y. (2023). Complications, adverse drug events, high costs, and disparities in multisystem inflammatory syndrome in children vs COVID-19. *JAMA Network Open, 6*(1), e2244975. https://doi.org/10.1001/jamanetworkopen.2022.44975

Eslami, K., Aletayeb, F., Aletayeb, S., Kouti, L., & Hardani, A. (2019). Identifying medication errors in neonatal intensive care units: A two-center study. *BMC Pediatrics, 19*(1), 365.

Fan, J., Jiang, Y., Hu, K., Chen, X., Xu, Q., et al. (2020). Barriers to using personal protective equipment by healthcare staff during the COVID-19 outbreak in China. *Medicine, 99*(48), e23310.

Gao, H., Li, Y., Jin, S., Zhai, W., Gao, Y., & Pu, L. (2024). Epidemiological characteristics and factors affecting healing in unintentional pediatric wounds. *Frontiers in Public Health, 12*, 1352176. https://doi.org/10.3389/fpubh.2024.1352176

Hsu, H. E., Mathew, R., Wang, R., Broadwell, C., Horan, K., Jin, R., Rhee, C., & Lee, G. M. (2020). Health care–associated infections among critically ill children in the US, 2013-2018. *JAMA Pediatrics, 174*(12), 1176–1183. https://doi.org/10.1001/jamapediatrics.2020.3223

Institute of Medicine. (2000). *To err is human: Building a safer health system.* National Academies Press.

Ladbrook, E., Khaw, D., Bouchoucha, S., & Hutchinson, A. (2021). A systematic scoping review of the cost-impact of ventilator-associated pneumonia (VAP) intervention bundles in intensive care. *American Journal of Infection Control, 49*(7), 928–936. https://doi.org/10.1016/j.ajic.2020.11.027

LeLaurin, J. H., & Shorr, R. I. (2019). Preventing falls in hospitalized patients: State of the science. *Clinical Geriatric Medicine, 35*(2), 273–283. https://doi.org/10.1016/j.cger.2019.01.007

Maryniak, K. (2019). *Professional nursing practice in the United States: An overview for international nurses, and those along the continuum from new graduates to experienced nurses.* Author.

Montastruc, J. L. (2023). Fatal adverse drug reactions in children: A descriptive study in the World Health Organization pharmacovigilance database. *British Journal of Clinical Pharmacology, 89*(1), 201–208. https://doi.org/10.1111/bcp.15470

Ottosen, M. J., Sedlock, E. W., Aigbe, A. O., Bell, S. K., Gallagher, T. H., & Thomas, E. J. (2021). Long-term impacts faced by patients and families after harmful healthcare events. *Journal of Patient Safety, 17*(8), e1145–e1151. https://doi.org/10.1097/PTS.0000000000000451

Ozeke, O., Ozeke, V., Coskun, O., & Budakoglu, I. I. (2019). Second victims in health care: Current perspectives. *Advances in Medical Education and Practice, 10*, 593–603.

Panagioti, M., Khan, K., Keers, R., Abuzour, A., & Phipps, D.,…& Ashcroft, D. (2019). Prevalence, severity, and nature of preventable patient harm across medical care settings: Systematic review and meta-analysis. *BMJ, 366*, l4185.

PSNet. (2019). *Medication errors and adverse drug events.* https://psnet.ahrq.gov/primer/medication-errors-and-adverse-drug-events

Salman, O., Procter, S., McGregor, C., Paul, P., Hutubessy, R., Lawn, J., Jit, Y., & M. (2020). Systematic review on the acute cost-of-illness of sepsis and meningitis in children and infants. *The Pediatric Infectious Disease Journal, 39*(1), 35–40.

Sentiff, J. L., Yenugadhati, V., Spitz, C., Glassman, S., Phillips, M., Frey, S., & Lesho, E. P. (2023). The impact of healthcare associated infections on costs and lengths of stay 2019–2023. *Open forum Infectious Diseases, 10*(Suppl 2), ofad500.2056. https://doi.org/10.1093/ofid/ofad500.2056

Shawahna, R., Jaber, M., Said, R., Mohammad, R., & Aker, Y. (2022). Medication errors in pediatric intensive care units: A multicenter qualitative study in the Palestinian practice. *BMC Pediatrics, 22*, 317.

Wang, H., Tsai, M., Chu, S., Liao, C., Lai, M., et al. (2021). Clinical characteristics and outcomes of children with polymicrobial ventilator-associated pneumonia in the intensive care unit. *BMC Infectious Diseases, 21*, 965.

Monitoring for and Detecting Nursing Errors

Identifying errors can be difficult and time-consuming. Most facilities have an event reporting system that is used to track and trend events once identified. It is more concerning that there are errors that go undetected or unreported due to fear of reprisal or punishment. It is important for facilities to adopt a safety program that is nonpunitive to encourage event reporting, a culture of open communication, transparency, and a quality assurance program that proactively monitors for abnormalities. Facilities should also have a strong internal audit program, including proactive risk assessments to help identify errors that may not be reported.

Nurses spend the majority of their time documenting and sometimes there is the thought that outcomes are improved through the act of documentation itself. Documentation is part of the process but should not be used to control a process. Nurses feel frustrated and overwhelmed with overcomplicated documentation that takes time away from the patient. Documentation should help guide the nurse but not be overly burdensome (Maryniak, 2021). Nurses need to spend their critical thinking skills on the patient assessment and needs, not on remembering all the nuances of documentation requirements.

Documentation should direct the nurse in telling the patient story in a way that the next caregivers understand what they need to provide good care (Maryniak, 2021). If nurses are struggling with documentation, then assessment of how the nursing documentation is set up must be done. The question should be asked if the documentation is set up in a way that helps guide the nurse to be successful and gives the appropriate information. If there are a lot of documentation errors or handoff events, the documentation templates should be examined.

A root cause analysis (RCA) is a process of working toward discovering the real cause of a problem. The focus is on resolving the actual cause rather than just looking at the symptoms of the issue. Contributing factors are identified during a discussion of the event. An RCA does not need to be done with every problem, as it is a time-consuming process. However, there are times when an RCA is required, such as with serious safety events (e.g., never events, or severe patient harm), repeat safety events, reportable patient injury (e.g., hospital-acquired conditions), a near miss with high potential for harm, family complaints, and at the discretion of leadership.

One method of analysis for an RCA is where a team looks at five "whys." In this method, the question "why" is asked repeatedly until the original reason for the error, also known as the root cause of a problem, is found (Maryniak, 2019). See also Fig. 5.1. A visual diagram, such as a fishbone, may be a useful tool to depict the contributing factors (see Fig. 5.2). Alternatively, the data about contributing factors from the RCA discussion can be listed in a table (see Fig. 5.3).

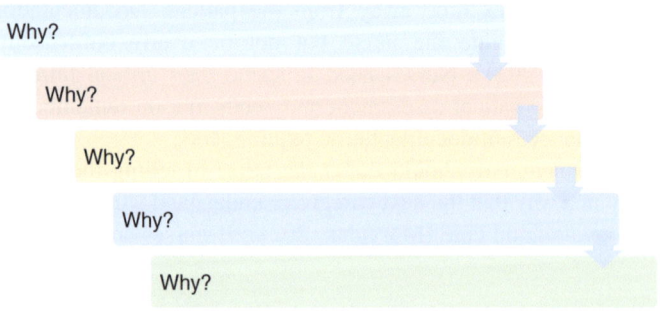

Fig. 5.1 Example of the "five whys"

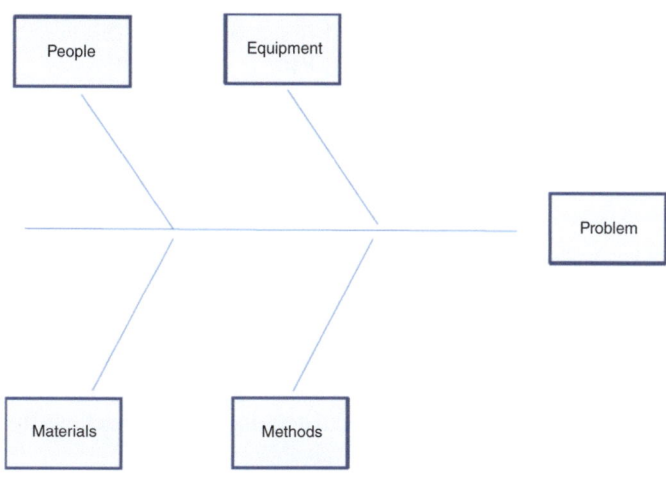

Fig. 5.2 Example of a fishbone diagram (Maryniak (2019). Used with permission)

Category	Contributing Factors
People	
Processes	
Equipment, supplies	
Culture	
Communication	
Staffing, training	

Fig. 5.3 Example of a contributing factors table

Many staff and leaders have been involved in root cause analysis or improvement plans. Following an RCA, a plan of corrective action should be developed. These plans should include measur-

Corrective Action	Measure of Success	Responsible Party	Due to Review

Fig. 5.4 Corrective action planning table

able and effective goals. An example of a table used for a corrective action is in Fig. 5.4. The key to making and sustaining actual improvement from an RCA is to determine goals and actions that are reasonable, actionable, and valuable.

Where there are errors, many times the first suggestions are to provide education and add some form of documentation audit. Those strategies are not generally effective, especially if the investigation and strategies do not get to the root cause of the error. And usually the audits are given to the nurses to perform, which takes away time spent with patients. To address issues and assist nurses, the processes and workspaces must be examined. Wastes must be reduced or eliminated from processes to help improve outcomes. Examples of waste can include time spent searching for supplies, overdocumentation, visual clutter, and constant interruptions. There is a term called "value added" in Lean Six Sigma for process steps (Maryniak, 2019). If a step doesn't add value, can't be done right the first time, and isn't something the customer is willing to pay for then that step should be eliminated, if possible.

If there are multiple errors found in a process that have different root causes, a good consideration would be to complete a Failure Modes and Effects Analysis (FMEA) to assess for vulnerability in the process. An FMEA can help identify vulnerable process steps, prioritize them by risk stratification, and implement mitigation strategies to decrease or eliminate the vulnerability (see also Fig. 5.5).

Failure Modes and Effects Analysis (FMEA) Form

Process/Product Name:

Problem:
Prepared by:

FMEA Date:

Severity (SEV): How severe is the effect on the customer? (5- most severe; 1- least severe)
Probability of Occurrence (OCC): How often does the cause occur? (5= highest occurrence; 1= lowest occurrence)
Detectability (DET): How well can you detect of the cause using the current controls? (5=most difficult to detect; 1= easily detected)
Risk Priority Number (RPN): What is the measure of process risk related to the effects, causes, & controls? (RPN + OCC+ DET)

Process Step/Input	Potential Failure Mode	Potential Failure Effects		Potential Causes		Current Controls			Action Recommended	Responsibility	Follow Up: Actions Taken				
			SEV		OCC		DET	RPN				Final SEV	Final OCC	Final DET	Final RPN
What is the process step under investigation?	What can go wrong with the process step/output?	What is the impact on the customer or internal requirements?		What are the root cause reasons for the process step/output to go wrong?		What are the existing controls that prevent or detect either the cause prior to leaving the process step?			What are the actions for reducing the OCC of the cause?	What is the target completion date and who is responsible?	What actions were completed and when?				
								0							0
								0							0
								0							0
								0							0
								0							0

Fig. 5.5 Example of an FMEA form

A culture of transparency and open communication is important to increase safety and decrease errors. This does not just happen; it must be planned and groomed. Many organizations that adopt lean principles use a type of daily management system to ensure open communication between frontline staff and leadership. This can be as simple as a white board used to communicate frontline needs and leadership expectations. Criteria is established to note the conditions for the shift, for example, if there needs to be adjustments to the workflow due to call offs, the number of patients in isolation, if there is equipment unavailable and staff need to be made aware so that they do not unnecessarily spend time looking for a piece of equipment that isn't available, etc. Leaders can use the board to help guide their rounding and to alert staff on new processes or process changes. The purpose is to improve safety and quality of care for patients by ensuring that those who care for the patients are well equipped, those who lead the caregivers are well informed, and ensure a connection to purpose.

An example of a daily management board includes the following information:

- Census, number of patients in isolation.
- Staffing available for the shift and on call staff available.
- Supplies that are on backorder, broken or missing equipment, and estimated time available.
- Identification of high-risk patients.
- New process, change in current process.

The caregivers can be better prepared for the shift and made aware of the department issues. The leaders can use the information to prioritize their rounding and monitor high-risk patients in the department. Leaders can have a bigger impact on safety if they assist in real time monitoring of high-risk patients and processes instead of the status quo of retrospective monitoring. Real time, concurrent monitoring with immediate feedback is more effective in process control and connecting the purpose (the "why") than retrospective monitoring. If problems are found days, weeks, or months after the fact, they are much harder to correct.

Using concurrent monitoring and mentoring can have an impact on the majority of healthcare associated infections and accidents. It is known that each day a child is intubated or has a central line in place, the chance of infection increases. Tightly controlled use of devices can decrease infection rates substantially. Education should focus on the dangers of using devices when they are not medically necessary, and why it is important to remove these as soon as possible (Letica-Kriegel et al., 2019). The daily management board can alert nurses and leaders about patients in the department with these devices to draw their attention for care and removal of the devices. Charge nurses can assess if the device is medically necessary and the leader can assess that the care is appropriate, providing real time feedback, to caregivers present, on any deviations noted. The old saying "it takes a village" applies to patient safety. It takes the entire team to keep patients safe. Tools such as a flowchart or value stream map can be useful to look at and evaluate the current state, and determine future states (see Figs. 5.6 and 5.7).

5 Monitoring for and Detecting Nursing Errors

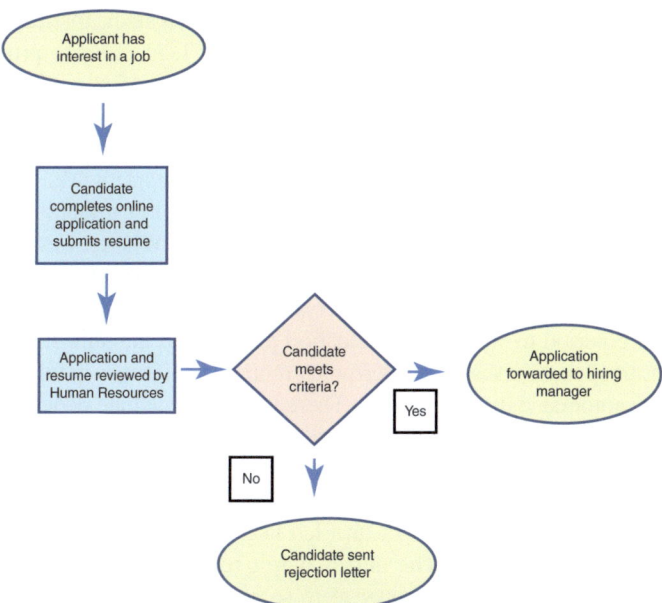

Fig. 5.6 Example of flowchart (Maryniak (2019). Used with permission)

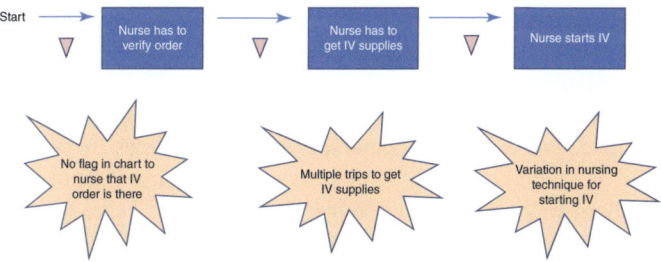

Fig. 5.7 Example of value stream analysis (Maryniak (2019). Used with permission)

The only way a nurse leader can assess what their nurses are spending their time on is by monitoring them where the work is happening. In Lean Six Sigma this is called going to the

Gemba —going to where the work happens (Kaizen Institute, n.d.). It is the responsibility of the nursing leadership to provide the tools and resources a nurse needs to provide a high quality of patient care. The only way to truly assess this is by going to where the work is being done and watching, asking questions, and seeing what works and what doesn't work.

An example of going to the Gemba occurred at a facility to help reduce medication errors in a pediatric unit. When reviewing the events, it was noted that there was a high number of errors at a specific time of the day. Observations were made during that time period to watch the medication pass within the unit. It was noticed that nurses were interrupted more than 30 times in total at the automated dispensing unit. There was an immediate review of the medication records, and several missed or delayed doses were found. This information was provided to the department director, and the location of the automated dispensing unit for this department was changed. This in turn led to a decrease in medication errors by over 50%. The nurses didn't realize they were interrupted so often because they were so used to getting disrupted. This was eye opening to the director and the nurses. Therefore, it is important for leaders to go where the work is and watch. The caregivers don't always recognize the factors contributing to errors because they develop a bias to them. Having fresh eyes on a situation can help find contributing factors that can be mitigated or even eliminated.

Standard work is also important to ensure that all caregivers complete processes in the same way and the outcomes are predictable. It would be very difficult to monitor a process if there is no standard way agreed on to complete the process. There are best practices available for many of the safety protocols, including monitoring and documentation. There should be standard expectations for care of high-risk patients that can be monitored easily by leadership. An example going back to indwelling central lines includes monitoring the care bundle. The caregivers should be aware of the best practices for caring for patients with central lines, including bundle elements for line insertion and maintenance. This information should be easy to understand and simple to monitor. If a process is not written down, it is not standard work.

Another concept of lean principles is mutual respect. Leaders are responsible for leading by example, managing up their peers and staff in a way that builds mutual respect. This further improves the culture of safety in facilities that is imperative for patient safety and high quality of care. When a leader focuses on processes and does not blame caregivers immediately for errors, caregivers are more likely to report errors because they feel safe to do so. Transparency is a two-way street when it comes to safety and high reliability. If the leaders make promises, it should be transparent to staff so they are held accountable for their actions as well.

Planning is essential, and considerations include the communication plan from frontline caregivers to leaders, and vice versa. Another question is how errors are handled, and if there is a culture of blame. Does the organization cultivate a culture of blame or does it look for cause, contributing factors, and process issues? Caregivers should know what is expected of them, and the leader's expectations must be clear with a connection to purpose. The organization needs to identify high-risk patients in departments, and staff must work as a team to care for these patients and ensure they are not further compromised. Processes should be easy to find and must be written in a way that all caregivers can understand and follow. Workarounds are due to poor processes or obstacles that continue to cause barriers and must be identified to make process improvements.

Other strategies to monitor for nursing errors include interdisciplinary rounding and leader rounding. Interdisciplinary rounding is valuable for nursing staff to ensure patient needs are met, which contributes to patient safety. Rounding on patients by nursing leaders is also helpful to focus on patient safety. Examples with children include ensuring bundles are in compliance (such as central line bundles), assessment of IV sites, and ensuring developmental care needs are met, such as environmental stimuli and supportive positioning (Maryniak, 2019).

Bedsides, nurses are also essential in identifying potential and actual errors. Catching errors before they occur or recognizing areas of opportunity with policies, procedures, and protocols can make a difference in current practices. With the increase in comorbidities and infections, it is important that nurses use tools to improve communication and transparency and ensure the work is standardized and easily accessible and understood.

References

Kaizen Institute. (n.d.). *Gemba and its meaning: The heart of lean management*. https://kaizen.com/insights/gemba-meaning-lean-management/

Letica-Kriegel, A. S., Salmasian, H., Vawdrey, D. K., Youngerman, B. E., Green, R. A., Furuya, E. Y., Calfee, D. P., & Perotte, R. (2019). Identifying the risk factors for catheter-associated urinary tract infections: A large cross-sectional study of six hospitals. *BMJ Open, 9*(2), e022137.

Maryniak, K. (2019). *Professional nursing practice in the United States: An overview for international nurses, and those along the continuum from new graduates to experienced nurses*. Author.

Maryniak, K. (2021). *Documentation for nurses* (4th ed.(ebook)). Elite Healthcare.

Best Practices to Prevent Nursing Errors

Scope of Practice

When looking at the potential for errors, nurses need to consider what is included in their nursing scope of practice. A scope of practice determines limitations and accountabilities of nurses. Although nursing scope of practice varies by location (such as state or province of licensure), there are some general common considerations included within the scope of practice. It is essential that nurses understand his or her scope of practice within their geographic location (e.g., state or province) (Maryniak, 2019).

Examples of limitations within a nursing scope of practice are that a nurse can only administer medications that are ordered by a licensed provider; nurses cannot order medications. Another practice consideration is that it is also beyond the scope of the nurse to medically diagnose (Maryniak, 2019). A provider may order protocols that identify specific circumstances and parameters for medication administration. Protocols may be implemented within an organization, which define circumstances or parameters for medication administration or other procedures. One example of a protocol that may be seen with pediatric patients is for nurse-driven catheter removal. Protocols are written for the criteria required to determine if an indwelling urinary catheter is required, or if it can be removed. If the criteria is not met, the nurse can remove the catheter per the protocol. These protocols also outline the ongoing assessment that is required for the catheter to remain out, such as bladder scans and the ability to void (AHRQ, 2020).

Nursing accountabilities within a scope of practice include that actions and interventions based on nursing assessment must either be ordered or included in policies, procedures, and protocols. This includes interventions that are part of medication administration. Nursing accountabilities include assessment, recognizing patient status changes, and using nursing judgment (Maryniak, 2019).

Bedside Report

Bedside report, also known as shift report or nursing handoff, is another effective strategy to help prevent errors. With bedside report, both the oncoming and off-going nurses participate in handoff at the bedside of the patient. The goal is to include the family in the report, which helps improve communication between staff and family. Research has shown that communication breakdown is correlated with adverse events (AHRQ, n.d.). Studies have also shown that bedside report increases family satisfaction, and does improve nursing satisfaction as well, when it is done effectively (Maryniak, 2019). Standardized bedside report can focus on safety, such as double checks with patient lines and equipment, activities, and plan of care. This interactive report can also assist in reinforcing family teaching (AHRQ, n.d.; Maryniak, 2019).

A recommended process for bedside report is as follows:

- Introduce the nursing staff to the family (if present) and invite them to participate in the bedside report.
- Access the health record.
- The off-going nurse will conduct a verbal report with the oncoming nurse and family (see standardized communication section below).
- Use words that the family can understand.
- The oncoming nurse will conduct a safety inspection of the room and a focused assessment of the patient.
  - Visually inspect all IV sites and tubing, wounds, etc.
  - Visually sweep the area for any physical safety concerns.

- Both nurses will review tasks that were done, or need to be done, such as:
  - Labs or tests needed.
  - Medications administered.
- Identify the patient's needs and family's needs or concerns, and discuss the goal(s).
- Some questions to ask the family may include:
  - "What could have gone better (during the shift)?"
  - "What concerns do you have?"
  - "What do you want to happen (during the next shift)?"
- Follow up to see if the goal was met during the next bedside report (AHRQ, n.d.).

Interdisciplinary Rounding

Rounding with pediatric patients looks very different than in the adult inpatient world, where purposeful patient rounding is routinely performed. Pediatric patient needs include regular safety checks, such as ensuring equipment is working appropriately, IV sites are assessed, patient comfort and positioning is assessed, and families are included. In addition to these basic needs, interdisciplinary rounding for bedside rounds is a best practice. Rounds at the bedside allow multiple disciplines to participate in reviewing patients and decision-making about care. Family members should also be included in bedside rounds, when possible, which increases their participation and improves transparency and communication. Studies have shown that interdisciplinary rounds increase patient safety as well as improve staff and family satisfaction rates (Cham et al., 2021; Shivananda et al., 2022).

A great interdisciplinary team requires respect, understanding of everyone's role, and effective communication. A team focus in addition to flexibility and vision assists with quality outcomes. The culture and relationships within a team should include recognition of each team member and their role and responsibility. Good communication in a team helps members feel that they are listened to and valued, and members should feel able to respectfully discuss and resolve issues within the group (Maryniak, 2019).

Standardized Communication

Standardized communication is essential in all aspects of healthcare. Effective communication between the interdisciplinary team and patients and families promote quality and safety. There are many formats for use in healthcare, whether it is for bedside report or discussing care with other team members, such as a provider. The most common one used is the SBAR, which stands for **S**ituation, **B**ackground, **A**ssessment, and **R**ecommendations. An explanation of the SBAR components are:

- Situation: This is a brief description of what is happening with the patient. This should include the current assessment and vital signs.
- Background: This includes the pertinent history of this patient, as it relates to the problem. This may contain diagnosis, medications, laboratory values, and interventions.
- Assessment: This is the assessment of the situation. Describe what the problem is at this time.
- Recommendations: This is any specific request about what the patient needs. Or, during report, this component may be the recommendation of what the patient needs (AHRQ, n.d.).

Another useful tool for standardized communication is the I-PASS, which stands for **I**llness severity, **P**atient summary, **A**ction list, **S**ituation awareness, and **S**ynthesis by receiver. Components of the I-PASS are:

- Illness severity: This is a description of how ill the patient is. This may also include code status.
- Patient summary: This is a brief patient overview, including pertinent information such as allergies, weight, hospital course, systems review (if there are concerns), and any pertinent history.
- Action list: This includes tasks that are pending, such as laboratory results, procedures, and medications.
- Situation awareness: This gives specific information about interventions or what may potentially go wrong. This will help the other person anticipate problems and be prepared.

- Synthesis by receiver: This allows for questions and clarifications to ensure that the information was received and understood (Blazin et al., 2020).

Strategies Specific to Infection Prevention

Nurses should be aware of the strategies to prevent contamination, particularly working with pediatric patients. This includes avoiding touching hands to face, and limiting touch of potentially contaminated surfaces. Standard precautions should be used judiciously with all patients, regardless of the level of isolation required (CDC, 2024). Hand hygiene should be performed frequently and efficiently. Times when hand hygiene should be performed include before entering a patient area, before touching a patient, prior to any aseptic procedures, after exposure to blood or body fluids, following touching a patient, after touching the patient environment, and after leaving the patient area. Gloves should also be replaced when heavily soiled or torn (CDC, n.d.). A commonly associated contributing cause of outbreaks of hospital-associated infections such as Clostridioides difficile (C. diff) or MDROs are organisms carried by the hands of nurses and other healthcare professionals (CDC, 2019).

Steps for handwashing are:

1. Wet hands with clean, running water (warm or cold), turn off the tap, and apply soap.
2. Lather hands by rubbing them together with the soap. Lather the backs of the hands, between the fingers, and under the nails.
3. Scrub hands for at least 20 s. Need a timer? Hum the "Happy Birthday" song from beginning to end twice.
4. Rinse hands well under clean, running water.
5. Dry hands using a clean towel or air dry them (see Fig. 6.1).

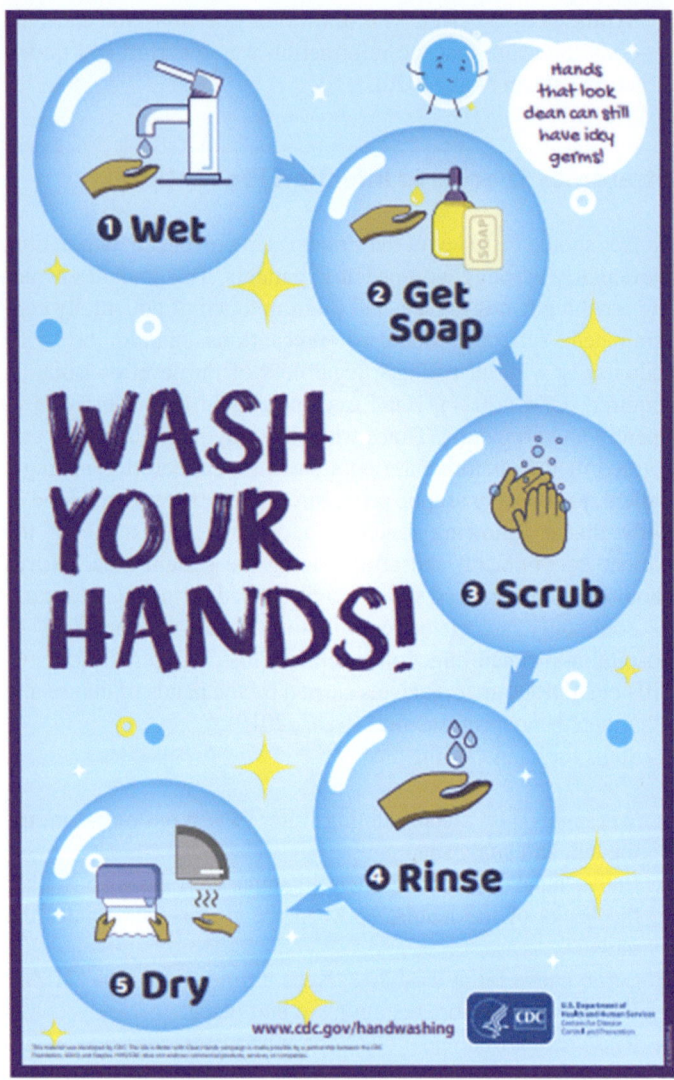

Fig. 6.1 Handwashing graphic. (Materials developed by CDC. https://www.cdc.gov/handwashing/pdf/wash-your-hands-poster-english2020-p.pdf. Reference to specific commercial products, manufacturers, companies, or trademarks does not constitute its endorsement or recommendation by the US Government, Department of Health and Human Services, or Centers for Disease Control and Prevention)

Strategies Specific to Infection Prevention

Steps for hand hygiene using alcohol-based hand rub (ABHR) are:

1. Apply the gel product to the palm of one hand (read the label to learn the correct amount).
2. Rub hands together.
3. Rub the gel over all the surfaces of hands and fingers until hands are dry. This should take around 20 s (see Fig. 6.2).

Understanding the PPE requirements for isolation and associated precautions is crucial. This includes communication and appropriate use of PPE in all areas of healthcare (CDC, 2019).

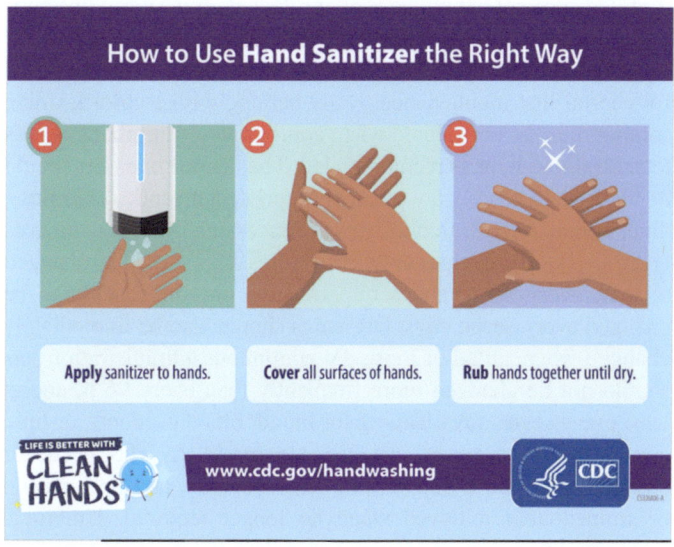

Fig. 6.2 Hand hygiene with ABHR graphic. (Materials developed by CDC. https://www.cdc.gov/handwashing/pdf/326806-A_Hand-Sanitizer-SignageSticker-Update-final2_11x8.5in_printonly.pdf. Reference to specific commercial products, manufacturers, companies, or trademarks does not constitute its endorsement or recommendation by the US Government, Department of Health and Human Services, or Centers for Disease Control and Prevention)

Approaches for Preventing CLABSIs

The best evidence for preventing CLABSIs include the use of bundles for both insertion and maintenance of central lines. For insertion, strategies include choosing the most appropriate insertion site based on the patient's needs, such as an umbilical venous catheter (UVC), tunneled catheter, or peripherally inserted central catheter (PICC). Hand hygiene and aseptic technique adherence is important prior to insertion. Maximal sterile barriers are required for line insertion. The central line insertion site should be prepared with chlorhexidine and alcohol solution when appropriate for gestational age and skin maturity. Closed systems should be used with standard precautions when accessing the devices. Prefilled syringes should be used for flushes, and central line antimicrobial locks may be considered (CDC, 2021a, b).

Effective hand hygiene and aseptic technique are also required for central line maintenance. Daily bathing with a chlorhexidine solution may be considered when appropriate. Minimizing access to central line hubs is recommended. The central line port should be vigorously scrubbed with an appropriate antiseptic (chlorhexidine, iodine, or 70% alcohol) prior to accessing. Access to devices is through sterile devices only. Gauze dressings should be changed at least every 48 h, and semipermeable dressings ought to be changed every seven days. Dressings should also be immediately changed when soiled or loose. IV continuous administration sets should not be changed more frequently than every 96 h, and at least every seven days. Tubing for blood, blood products, or lipid administration requires changing every 24 h. The need for continuing a central line is to be assessed daily, and lines should be immediately removed when no longer required. Umbilical lines should be removed within seven days (CDC, 2021a, b).

Best Practices for Avoiding CAUTIs

CAUTIs can occur with prolonged use of an indwelling urinary catheter, particularly with at risk patients such as elderly, immunocompromised, or female. Use of a CAUTI prevention bundle can be effective in reducing the risk. The most effective strategy is to avoid insertion of an indwelling catheter unless absolutely necessary, and removing them as soon as possible. Indications for indwelling catheters may be for urinary retention (if a bladder protocol is not effective), as required by a urologist, or comfort care. Use of indwelling catheters for surgery should be limited and removed as soon as able postoperatively. Patients in intensive care units do not require routine use of indwelling catheters (Triplett et al. 2021).

Hand hygiene and aseptic technique are vital during catheter insertion and during catheter care. It is recommended to use closed, preconnected catheter systems. Other strategies as part of a bundle include assessing and avoiding kinking of the catheter and tubing, ensuring the collection bag is below the level of the bladder, and confirming the bag is not on the floor. Regular cleansing of the catheter and perineum are also needed. Ongoing assessment of the catheter and determination for ongoing use is also essential. Many organizations have a policy for use of a nurse-driven catheter removal protocol which, if used appropriately, can remove the catheter in a timelier fashion (Triplett et al., 2021).

Preventing Ventilator-Associated Pneumonia

Ventilator bundles are designed to prevent VAP, but the main initiative against preventing any VAE is to minimize the time the patient is on the ventilator. Strategies include using alternatives to intubation, assessing the need for ventilation daily, and weaning off the ventilator as soon as possible. Weaning from sedation is also important, and use of spontaneous awakening with breathing trials is indicated. Prevention also includes hand hygiene, suctioning only as needed, and use of histamine 2 receptor antagonists or antacids. Oral antimicrobials may be used along with probiotics. Other strategies include providing good oral care frequently with an antiseptic solution. Maintaining elevation of the head of the bed, when appropriate, can prevent aspiration. Use of low tidal volumes and conservative fluid management are also good approaches (Klompas, 2019).

Strategies for Preventing Pressure Injuries

Pressure injuries, also known as bedsores, pressure ulcers, or decubitus ulcers, are damage that occur to the skin and soft tissues. Prolonged pressure, friction, shear, and poor nutritional status can predispose patients to developing pressure injuries. Pressure injuries may or may not be associated with pain. Pediatric patients are at risk for pressure injuries due to immature skin, disease processes, compromised circulation, procedures and surgery, prolonged sitting or time in bed, incontinence, medical devices, and pressure on bony prominences (Haesler, 2019).

Performing comprehensive skin assessments is essential to identify patients at risk for pressure injury followed by implementation of individualized prevention plans. Standardized risk assessment tools should be used, and the skin should be assessed frequently. The entire skin from head to toe should be examined for abnormalities and injury. This requires visualization under clothes with particular focus on body prominences, and under medical devices (Broom et al., 2019; Haesler, 2019).

The skin should be compared symmetrically, noting any differences in skin color, temperature, or areas that do not blanch. Moisture, skin turgor, and skin integrity should be assessed. If wounds or discoloration is noted, this should be documented and photographed (Maryniak, 2021).

Staff knowledge of the potential for skin damage and gentle handling is essential for the prevention of skin injury. Employees' nails should be short and gloves used for handling. Equipment and supplies can create injury, including the use of adhesives. Minimizing use of equipment to essentials, nominal use of adhesives, removal of any additional supplies within the bed, appropriate cleaning of the child, and frequent positioning with developmental support are also needed (Broom et al., 2019).

Fall Prevention Strategies

Patient assessment is a priority to identify patients at risk for falling, and implementing individualized strategies to help prevent falls. Use of a standardized fall assessment tool is needed, which identifies risk factors for falling. Examples of risk factors include age, difficulty ambulating or transferring, frequent toileting needs, history of previous falls, medications, sensory impairment, alterations in mental status, and medical conditions (LeLaurin & Shorr, 2019).

All patients should have standard fall precautions, such as orienting the patient to the room environment and call light, ensuring personal items and call light are within reach, and placing hospital beds in the lowest position while the patient is in bed. Brakes should be on hospital beds, chairs, and wheelchairs when stationary. Nonslip well-fitted footwear, such as socks, should be provided to patients. Appropriate lighting, including the use of night lights, and sturdy handrails in rooms, bathrooms, and halls are needed. Environments should be clean and clutter-free, with clean, dry floors. Safe patient handling techniques are essential when assisting patients, including the use of a gait belt when ambulating patients. Purposeful rounding on a regular basis can also assist in meeting patient needs and assessing safety, including measures for fall prevention (LeLaurin & Shorr, 2019; Maryniak, 2019).

Additional safety precautions are required for patients at risk for falls. These should be individualized to the patient. Interventions for risk factors should be implemented, such as supervising and reorienting patients with cognitive impairment, assessing medication effects, and creating a safe environment. Patients at high risk, particularly those with cognitive impairment and impulsivity, may require the use of a sitter to constantly monitor patient activity. The use of tele sitters is an alternative, but this is not recommended for patients who have altered mental status or cognitive impairment. Medication effects should be assessed by nurses, pharmacists, and providers to determine if there are alternatives, which may decrease fall risk. Monitoring of patient vital signs and slow transitions to ambulating are essential if patient medication increases fall risk. Impairment in mobility may require use of assistive devices, which should be easily accessible. Use of transfer devices or lifts may be necessary for safe patient handing (LeLaurin & Shorr, 2019).

Education of the patient and family, including the use of signs to remind them to ask for assistance with ambulating, may be effective. Bed and chair alarms may also remind the patient to wait for help, but they are not an effective strategy for impulsive patients. Many times, the alarm may not be heard by staff until the patient is already out of the bed or chair (LeLaurin & Shorr, 2019).

Many organizations have fall prevention programs which include the use of visual cues for the interdisciplinary team. Use of colored signs, socks, and wristbands can alert all team members that a patient is a fall risk (LeLaurin & Shorr, 2019).

Strategies for Preventing Medication Errors

When reviewing strategies to prevent medication errors, there are those at a system level to consider. The National Patient Safety Goals, developed by the Joint Commission, are used as standards for patient safety at organizations throughout the United States. The goals are developed around areas that can be problems in healthcare and are a focus of safety. The 2025 goals include correct patient identification and safe medication use. Other categories focus on improving interdisciplinary clinical communication, reducing patient harm associated with clinical alarms, reducing risks of hospital-acquired infections, and identifying patient safety risks (The Joint Commission, 2025).

There are multiple strategies at the system level to help decrease the chance for medication errors, which should be incorporated in organizational processes. The use of two patient identifiers, such as name and date of birth, must be used with medication administration. All medications should be labeled, such as those in syringes or other containers. Anticoagulants, such as blood thinners, put patients at higher risk for complications. Extra care and assessment should be practiced with these patients. Maintaining medication reconciliation is important throughout the patient's continuum, including transition from hospital to home, and with every outpatient visit (The Joint Commission, 2025).

Another important focus for system improvement is policies and procedures, such as those involving medication administration. These should be developed based on evidence, and must meet regulatory and accreditation standards. Multidisciplinary team members provide key stakeholders who are involved in medication administration. Shared governance is effective by adding frontline staff who can add valuable insight into policies. Staff buy-in is also improved when they are part of the process, including policy development. Policies differ from guidelines in that they must be followed. Education about policies includes this fact, and staff need to be held accountable for following policies. Organizations should clearly define reporting processes for medication errors. This may include verbal reporting, such as to a provider, and written or electronic reporting processes. Policies for security and access regarding medications should also be created for facilities. This includes requirements for secured location of medication, and which employees are authorized to access medications (such as licensed personnel). Medication administration policies may also include the use of technology, such as bar-coded medication administration, computerized provider order entry, and smart IV pumps (Hanson & Haddad, 2023).

Other policy and procedure considerations include safety standards. Organizations should define unacceptable abbreviations. The Joint Commission (n.d.) has a list of unacceptable abbreviations, and the Institute for Safe Medication Practices (ISMP) also has an extended list of abbreviations, symbols, and other written information, which can potentially cause medical errors (ISMP, 2021). Unacceptable abbreviations must be defined within a facility. Reference lists are available through the Joint Commission and the Institute for Safe Medication Practices. Examples of unacceptable abbreviations include:

- Avoiding "u" and spelling out "units".
- Avoiding "IU" and spelling out "international units".
- Writing out "daily" and "every other day" rather than using "qd," and "qod".
- Not using trailing 0 after a decimal point.
- Using 0 before a decimal point.
- Writing out morphine sulfate or magnesium sulfate rather than abbreviating with "ms".
- Using "mL" rather than cc.
- Writing out "discharge" or "discontinue" rather than using the "d/c" abbreviation (ISMP, 2021; The Joint Commission, n.d.).

High risk medications should be defined within the organization and practices related to high-risk medication also require documentation. Strategies to decrease risk of medication errors with high-risk medications (ISMP, 2018) include:

- Standardization of ordering, storage, preparation, and administration of these medications.
- Improved access to information about these drugs.
- Access to high-alert medications should be limited.
- Supplementary labels and automated alerts can be used.
- Use of redundancies, such as independent double checks.

The ISMP (2018) also has a list of recommended high-risk medications, identified as those which can cause significant patient harm. These include classes of:

- Adrenergic agonists, IV (e.g., epinephrine, phenylephrine, norepinephrine).
- Adrenergic antagonists, IV (e.g., propranolol, metoprolol, labetalol).

Strategies for Preventing Medication Errors

- Anesthetic agents, general, inhaled and IV (e.g., propofol, ketamine).
- Antiarrhythmics, IV (e.g., lidocaine, amiodarone).
- Antithrombotic agents, including: anticoagulants (e.g., warfarin, low molecular weight heparin, unfractionated heparin); direct oral anticoagulants and factor Xa inhibitors (e.g., dabigatran, rivaroxaban, apixaban, edoxaban, betrixaban, fondaparinux); direct thrombin inhibitors (e.g., argatroban, bivalirudin, dabigatran); glycoprotein IIb/IIIa inhibitors (e.g., eptifibatide); thrombolytics (e.g., alteplase, reteplase, tenecteplase).
- Cardioplegic solutions.
- Chemotherapeutic agents, both parenteral and oral.
- Dextrose, hypertonic, 20% or greater.
- Dialysis solutions, both peritoneal and hemodialysis.
- Epidural and intrathecal medications.
- Inotropic medications, IV (e.g., digoxin, milrinone).
- Insulin, subcutaneous and IV.
- Liposomal forms of drugs (e.g., liposomal amphotericin B) and conventional counterparts (e.g., amphotericin B desoxycholate).
- Moderate sedation agents, IV (e.g., dexmedetomidine, midazolam, lorazepam).
- Moderate and minimal sedation agents, oral, for children (e.g., chloral hydrate, midazolam, ketamine [using the parenteral form]).
- Opioids, including: IV; oral (including liquid concentrates, immediate- and sustained-released formulations); transdermal.
- Neuromuscular blocking agents (e.g., succinylcholine, rocuronium, vecuronium).
- Parenteral nutrition preparations.
- Sodium chloride for injection, hypertonic, greater than 0.9% concentration.
- Sterile water for injection, inhalation and irrigation (excluding pour bottles) in containers of 100 mL or more.
- Sulfonylurea hypoglycemics, oral (e.g., chlorpropamide, glimepiride, glyburide, glipizide, tolbutamide).

Specific medications identified as high-risk are:

- Epinephrine, IM, subcutaneous.
- Epoprostenol (e.g., Flolan), IV.
- Insulin U-500 (special emphasis*) (*All forms of insulin, subcutaneous and IV, are considered a class of high-alert medications. Insulin U-500 has been singled out for special emphasis to bring attention to the need for distinct strategies to prevent the types of errors that occur with this concentrated form of insulin).
- Magnesium sulfate injection.
- Methotrexate, oral, non-oncologic use.
- Nitroprusside sodium for injection.
- Opium tincture.
- Oxytocin, IV.
- Potassium chloride for injection concentrate.
- Potassium phosphates injection.
- Promethazine injection.
- Vasopressin, IV and intraosseous.

Another system consideration for decreasing medication errors is staff resources. Access to expert human resources on medications is needed, such as pharmacists. Medication supplies can be immediately available through unit stock or medication storage, such as electronic dispensaries. Staff need access to medication information, through either a current version of pharmacology textbooks or electronic access, such as online databases or apps. Equipment needed for medication administration should be working and accessible. Examples include IV or syringe pumps, syringes and other supplies, and bar-coded medication technology (Hanson & Haddad, 2023).

Education, training, the work environment, and culture are other system considerations. Both education and experiences help to increase familiarity with commonly used medications. Didactic education for nurses is one strategy, such as inclusion in new graduate nurse residency programs. Clinical experiences include preceptorships with skilled staff to assist knowledge attainment.

Work confidence through orientation to the environment can also assist. This can improve time management and decrease stress levels.

Appropriate staffing and workload are common struggles in organizations. Many organizations use ratio-based nursing, which does not consider patient acuity or level of skill of staff. Nurses who are in orientation or preceptorship should not be given full assignments until appropriate. The skill mix needs to consider licensed and unlicensed personnel. Additionally, staffing should consider how many experienced and inexperienced nurses are working during a shift.

Physical environments can impact on staff stress and well-being. These can also create distractions from the environment itself. Distractions and interruptions, as common identified contributors to errors, must be minimized. Some strategies include use of safe zones that are physically identified in medication rooms or around automated medication dispensaries. Other indicators to limit distractions are the use of tags to identify when a nurse is administering medications. Staff should also be empowered to safely state that he or she must focus on medication administration.

Supervision is a consideration for newer nurses in particular, when they are learning skills around medication administration. Supportive work environments are those where nurses feel empowered, and participate in shared governance. Team work is important to help one another learn and grow, and meet the needs of patients and families. Instituting a just culture is also essential. Visible, supportive leaders who have good relationships with staff create a positive work environment. There must be trust between staff and leaders, which increases an effective culture. Fear or distrust decreases the chance that errors are effectively reported, and therefore processes are not evaluated (Rodziewicz et al., 2021).

System considerations about the use of technology is also needed. As we grow in the use of technology in healthcare, it is important to understand that it is an additional tool to assist staff, but cannot replace critical thinking. Nurses are the last stop to safety with medication administration, and so complacency with technology can be dangerous. Bar coded medication administration is an important strategy for medication safety. However, not all errors are caught with this technology. For example, if a nurse is to administer a partial dose, it is up to that nurse to appropriately administer the correct dose, like in the case of insulin. Additionally, the technology will not necessarily identify when a medication should not be given (such as holding a beta blocker if heart rate or blood pressure is outside parameters). Smart IV pumps are programmed with drug libraries as well as dose reduction systems (which assists with preventing inadvertent high doses). Nurse diligence can assist in identifying and verifying dosages. In one case, new IV pumps were programmed for an incorrect concentration of a medication in one facility. A nurse was verifying calculations and caught the error quickly. As a result of her diligence, all of the pumps at the facility were immediately reprogrammed with the right medication concentration.

Just as personal health and stress are correlated with medication errors, personal wellness is associated with better outcomes, and reduced chance for errors. Staff need to ensure that they are getting adequate rest at home and taking breaks at work. It is also important not only to identify areas of stress but also address the stress, such as the use of coping mechanisms. Staff also need to stay home from work if ill (Rodziewicz et al., 2021).

Nurses must follow the rights of medication administration each and every time. The five basic rights of medication administration are right patient, drug, time, dose, and route. Throughout the years, additional rights have been discussed, up to 12 rights in total, such as right reason, education, documentation, right to refusal and expiration date. However, the five basic rights are consistently recommended. Nurses are also accountable to following policies and procedures. If there is unfamiliarity with policies, then referring to them should be done until familiar. Nurses should never give any medication without knowing the reason, possible side effects, interactions, safe dose range, monitoring, etc. (Rodziewicz et al., 2021).

Nurses as advocates can assist the family with effective teaching, and encouraging them to speak up if there are any concerns or if they do not understand something. Nurses must also listen to concerns. For example, if a family states "Oh, the doctor said he was going to stop giving my baby that medication," then the nurse should verify before either administering or holding a medication. Promoting self-wellness and a supportive work culture assists everyone, including patients and families (Maryniak, 2019).

Using a Daily Management System

As discussed in Chap. 5, use of a daily management system (DMS) can increase awareness, improve communication, foster transparency, help reduce errors, and improve safety. Daily management allows staff doing the work and leaders at all levels of the organization to clearly visualize whether the performance is on track (no variations) or has deviated from target condition(s). Some key points about DMS are:

- A DMS helps to rapidly identify deviation and correct the problem by bringing attention to the problem and quickly addressing the cause.
- Everyone has equal responsibility for taking necessary actions to quickly correct the problem or escalate as needed.
- Old school of thought brought attention to the problem after the fact making it difficult to find causation and fix; DMS brings immediate attention with expectation to address causation or escalate barriers as needed.

One example is focus on reducing CLABSIs. A system goal would be zero harm, with a facility goal of reducing CLABSI events. The department goal would then be decreasing the indwelling central line catheter days (see Fig. 6.3).

The dwell time has the highest impact on developing CLABSIs—each day increases the chance of infection. Therefore, if the dwell time can be reduced then CLABSIs can also be decreased. The room number of patients with central lines would be placed on the DMS boards, and these patients would be prioritized in leader and interdisciplinary rounding to ensure they meet the criteria for the line or it is removed. The same principle would be used for hospital acquired pressure injuries (HAPIs) as well (see Table 6.1).

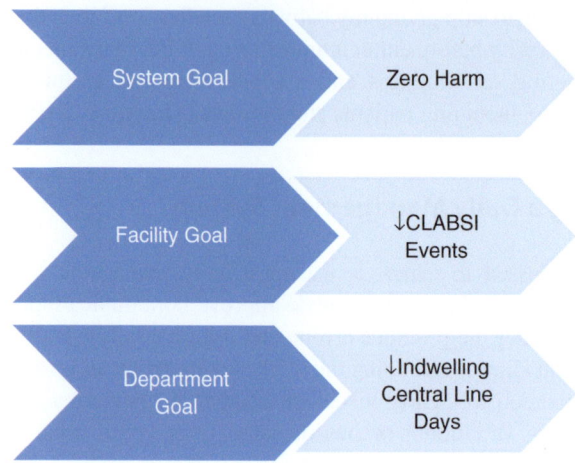

Fig. 6.3 Alignment of goals

Table 6.1 Example of process monitoring on DMS board

Outcome metric	# since last huddle	Days since last incidence	Process metric today	Comments
Central lines	5	N/A	N/A	Beds 1, 14, 16, 22, 24
CLABSI	0	250	100%	Bundle compliance goal 95%
Skin injury	0	22	100%	
Ventilators	6	N/A	N/A	Beds 1, 2, 14, 16, 22, 24
VAP	0	165	95%	Bundle compliance goal 95%
Hand hygiene	N/A	N/A	75%	Bundle compliance goal 95%

It is important to prioritize rounding and monitoring to aid in reduction of harm events. Whenever a patient has a device, they should be monitored closely to ensure the device is needed, and if so, the correct processes involved with care of the device are strictly adhered to. The only way to effectively monitor this is by making this a priority.

References

Agency for Healthcare Research and Quality (AHRQ). (2020). Appendix M. Example of a nurse-driven protocol for catheter removal. https://www.ahrq.gov/hai/cauti-tools/impl-guide/implementation-guide-appendix-m.html

Agency for Healthcare Research and Quality (AHRQ). (n.d.). *Nurse bedside shift report: Implementation handbook.* https://www.ahrq.gov/sites/default/files/wysiwyg/professionals/systems/hospital/engagingfamilies/strategy3/Strat3_Implement_Hndbook_508.pdf

Blazin, L. J., Sitthi-Amorn, J., Hoffman, J. M., & Burlison, J. D. (2020). Improving patient handoffs and transitions through adaptation and implementation of I-PASS across multiple handoff settings. *Pediatric Quality & Safety, 5*(4), e323.

Broom, M., Dunk, A., Mohamed, E., & A. (2019). Predicting pediatric skin injury: The first step to reducing skin injuries in children. *Health Service Insights, 14*, 12.

Centers for Disease Control & Prevention. (2019). *2007 guideline for isolation precautions: Preventing transmission of infectious agents in healthcare settings* (updated 2019). https://www.cdc.gov/infectioncontrol/pdf/guidelines/isolation-guidelines-H.pdf.

Centers for Disease Control & Prevention. (2024). *Multidrug-resistant organisms (MDRO) management guidelines.* https://www.cdc.gov/infectioncontrol/hcp/mdro-management/index.html.

Centers for Disease Control & Prevention. (n.d.). *Sequence for putting on personal protective equipment (PPE).* https://www.cdc.gov/hai/pdfs/ppe/ppe-sequence.pdf

Centers for Disease Control and Prevention (CDC). (2021a). *NICU: CLABSI guidelines.* https://www.cdc.gov/infectioncontrol/guidelines/nicu-clabsi/index.html.

Centers for Disease Control and Prevention (CDC). (2021b). *Outbreak investigations in healthcare settings.* https://www.cdc.gov/hai/outbreaks/index.html

Cham, P., Ellsworth, L., Gisondo, C., Lawrence, C., & Weiner, G. (2021). An analysis of neonatal intensive care daily rounds in a level IV unit. *Pediatrics, 147*(3_MeetingAbstract), 420–421.

Haesler, E. (Ed.). (2019). *Prevention and treatment of pressure ulcers/injuries: The international guideline 2019.* Cambridge Media.

Hanson, A., & Haddad, L. M. (2023). *Nursing rights of medication administration.* StatPearls Publishing. https://www.ncbi.nlm.nih.gov/books/NBK560654/

Institute for Safe Medication Practices. (2018). *High alert medications in acute care settings.* https://www.ismp.org/recommendations/high-alert-medications-acute-list

Institute for Safe Medication Practices. (2021). *ISMP'S list of error-prone abbreviations, symbols, and dose designations.* https://www.ismp.org/Tools/errorproneabbreviations.pdf

Klompas, M. (2019). Ventilator-associated events: What they are and what they are not. *Respiratory Care, 64*(8), 953–961. https://doi.org/10.4187/respcare.07059

LeLaurin, J. H., & Shorr, R. I. (2019). Preventing falls in hospitalized patients: State of the science. *Clinical Geriatric Medicine, 35*(2), 273–283. https://doi.org/10.1016/j.cger.2019.01.007

Maryniak, K. (2019). *Professional nursing practice in the United States: An overview for international nurses, and those along the continuum from new graduates to experienced nurses.* Author.

Maryniak, K. (2021). *Documentation for nurses* (4th ed. (ebook)). Elite Healthcare.

Rodziewicz, T. L., Houseman, B., & Hipskind, J. E. (2021). Medical error reduction and prevention. In *StatPearls*. StatPearls Publishing. https://pubmed.ncbi.nlm.nih.gov/29763131/

Shivananda, S., Osiovich, H., de Salaberry, J., Hait, V., & Gautham, K. (2022). Improving efficiency of multidisciplinary bedside rounds in the NICU: A single Centre QI project. *Pediatric Quality & Safety, 7*(1), e511.

The Joint Commission. (2025). *2025 hospital National Patient Safety Goals.* https://www.jointcommission.org/-/media/tjc/documents/standards/national-patient-safety-goals/2025/hap-npsg-simplified-2025-accessible.pdf.

The Joint Commission. (n.d.). *Facts about the official "Do Not Use" list of abbreviations.* https://www.jointcommission.org/resources/news-and-multimedia/fact-sheets/facts-about-do-not-use-list/

Triplett, A., Zeller, K., & Potisek, N. (2021). Indwelling lines. *Pediatric Review, 42*(2), 106–108. https://doi.org/10.1542/pir.2020-002303

Case Studies

Case Study #1

Casey was a two-year-old female admitted to the pediatric unit yesterday with bronchiolitis from respiratory syncytial virus (RSV). On night shift the nurse noted that Casey had redness and wateriness in both eyes. Casey was also rubbing her eyes.

Two days later, the patient in the next bed, Joseph, was also noted to have watery, red eyes. Joseph was a five-year-old male admitted with acute asthma exacerbation. The same day that Joseph developed the symptoms, another patient in the unit, Lily, developed the same symptoms. Lily was an eight-year-old female with diabetic ketoacidosis.

The charge nurse identified the trend with the patients' signs and symptoms, and called the infection preventionist. All three patients were placed in contact plus standard precautions. The provider took cultures from the three patients, which were positive for bacterial conjunctivitis.

The nursing manager, risk manager, and infection preventionist determined that a root cause analysis would be warranted in this situation. They invited nurses, providers, and respiratory therapists to the RCA.

- In reviewing the spread of conjunctivitis amongst the patients, why did this happen?

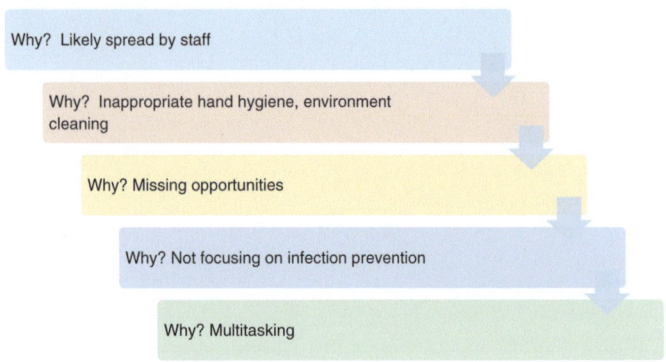

Fig. 7.1 RCA for case study #1 with the "five whys"

The group participating in the RCA, using the five whys, determined the contributing factors involved (see Fig. 7.1).

The RCA group discussed that there were appropriate processes in place, through policies and procedures, about hand hygiene and environmental cleaning. They also identified that there were appropriate equipment and supplies available for hand hygiene and environmental cleaning. The staff determined that the most likely cause of the cases of conjunctivitis was spread through staff. This finding aligns with statements from the CDC that outbreaks often occur from a failure to uphold infection prevention and control practices (CDC, 2021). The group admitted that there were missed opportunities for both hand hygiene and environmental cleaning amongst staff, including themselves. Examples included not changing gloves and performing hand hygiene when working from dirty to clean, not always performing hand hygiene at each opportunity (especially if there was a sense of urgency between patients), and not cleaning the environment (such as counters or bedside tables) with every opportunity. These behaviors were identified as at-risk, using a just culture process. Contributing factors also included the need to reinforce infection prevention practices, hold staff accountable to these practices, and communicate results from infection prevention audits (see Table 7.1).

Findings from the RCA were shared with the leadership, and a corrective action plan was created to be implemented within the department (see Table 7.2).

Table 7.1 Contributing factors for case study #1

Category	Contributing factors
People	Missing opportunities for hand hygiene and environmental cleaning; not focusing
Processes	Processes for hand hygiene and cleaning were in place
Equipment, supplies	Equipment and supplies were available
Culture	Need reinforcement of accountability for hand hygiene, appropriate use of PPE, environmental cleaning
Communication	Communication of hand hygiene audits were not done with staff
Staffing, training	Need to reinforce hand hygiene, PPE, and environmental cleaning practices

Table 7.2 Corrective action plan for case study #1

Corrective action	Measure of success	Responsible party	Due to review
Reeducate staff on infection prevention measures, including reinforcing appropriate hand hygiene, use of PPE, and environmental cleaning practices	Staff will successfully pass a posttest with a minimum of 80%	Clinical education	One month
Hand hygiene audits will be performed and results will be shared with the staff	Audits will show 95% compliance with hand hygiene 100% of results will be posted on DMS board and reviewed with all staff	Infection prevention	Monthly
Managers will reinforce accountability for infection prevention practices, including hand hygiene, appropriate use of PPE, environmental cleaning with staff	Infection prevention practices will be documented in staff performance reviews Progressive discipline, if warranted based on just culture, will occur for not following infection prevention practices	Managers	Ongoing

Case Study #2

A nurse leader, Ronald, was rounding on the unit and saw a new nurse Samantha (who was just off orientation) performing a central line dressing change on her own. The patient was a 10-month-old male. The policy and procedure in the pediatric unit was to have two staff at the bedside to perform sterile procedures, including changing the dressing with central lines. Ronald also noted that Samantha contaminated the new dressing as she was preparing to place it on the patient.

Ronald joined Samantha at the bedside and stopped the procedure, and had her start over, with Ronald assisting. Ronald walked Samantha through the procedure and helped her maintain sterility throughout.

After completion of the procedure, Ronald had a private conversation with Samantha and asked her what education she had been given for performing central line dressing changes. Samantha stated she had only participated in a sterile dressing change once, and tried to follow what her preceptor was doing. She also said that she only had one opportunity to practice sterile technique in a skills lab during her nursing school. Samantha was not aware that she had broken sterile technique, or that two people were needed for the procedure. Ronald identified that this was a human error, and that Samantha needed more education and reinforcement. Ronald spoke with Samantha about the importance of following the policy and procedure, and to have knowledge of sterile techniques.

Ronald also realized that Samantha's preceptor, Joel, might need more information, and so he spoke with him. Ronald learned that Joel had very little experience with central line dressing changes since he had just been transferred from a lower level of pediatric care, where central lines were used infrequently. Joel stated that his orientation had felt rushed, and there were learning opportunities for him as well.

Ronald worked with the educator, and they revised the orientation for new nurses to include simulation with sterile technique. Preceptor education was also revised based on the feedback. Communications with staff were done, reminding them of where policies and procedures were located. Additionally, competencies were developed for sterile technique and central line dressing changes. Monthly audits were instituted following education, which showed an increase in compliance with sterile technique and central line maintenance, including dressing changes.

Summary

The case studies provide actual examples of errors that have occurred in pediatric care. They demonstrate how to identify errors and processes for evaluating the errors through communication and use of tools. These cases also show how to make improvements through improving processes, education, and communication.

Reference

Centers for Disease Control and Prevention (CDC). (2021). *Outbreak investigations in healthcare settings.* https://www.cdc.gov/hai/outbreaks/index.html

Recommendations for Further Study

8

It has been noted that there are studies that examine various errors in nursing and in healthcare. The frequency of errors directly related to pediatric patients is not commonly seen in the literature. For example, there are many studies which examine adult hospital-acquired conditions such as CLABSI, CAUTI, and VAP, but not as many looking specifically at conditions in the pediatric population (Speer et al., 2023). Additionally, studies regarding errors have mainly focused on medication errors. There are opportunities in the literature to further delve into pediatric-specific conditions and nursing practices. This should be done in all pediatric settings, including different levels of pediatric intensive care and acute care settings. Errors in pediatric ambulatory settings such as clinics or follow up programs in the home can also be examined.

Pediatric patients are very specialized, and the level of acuity can vary from healthy to acutely ill. More examination of environmental contributing factors that can lead to errors may be warranted. The work environment, stress, additional time constraints, and current changes in the workforce can increase the risk of errors with pediatric patients. There may also be additional stacking in the minds of nurses caring for these patients, which can also lead to errors. There are opportunities to further delve into specific system and personal contributing factors for errors. Examining organizational traits, including staffing practices, use of skill mix, and incorporation of best practices into policies and procedures compared with error rates, can provide valuable information. Looking at personal considerations, including years of experience, education, certification, and leader qualities correlating with rates of errors is also needed (Manias et al., 2021).

Examining personal effects of errors from the perspective of the family and the nurse is also required. Both quantitative and qualitative studies would add significance to this topic.

References

Manias, E., Street, M., Lowe, G., Low, J. K., Gray, K., & Botti, M. (2021). Associations of person-related, environment-related and communication-related factors on medication errors in public and private hospitals: A retrospective clinical audit. *BMC Health Services Research, 21*, 1025. https://doi.org/10.1186/s12913-021-07033-8

Speer, E. M., Lee, L. K., Bourgeois, F. T., Gitterman, D., Hay, W. W., Jr., Davis, J. M., & Javier, J. R. (2023). The state and future of pediatric research: An introductory overview. *Pediatric Research.* https://doi.org/10.1038/s41390-022-02439-4

Summary

Caring for pediatric patients requires complex nursing care. Baseline knowledge about common pediatric conditions is essential for nursing staff. There are errors that can occur related to nursing care, such as inappropriate or omitted hand hygiene, medication errors, or hospital-acquired conditions. Errors with a child can create life-long consequences.

There are multiple factors that can contribute to nursing errors, both at system and personal levels. Together, organizations, leaders, and staff are accountable for ensuring there are appropriate processes for reducing the risk of errors. Diligence, communication, and a constant focus on safety is required.

Potential or actual errors can create a near-miss situation, or one with actual harm. Consequences of nursing errors can be detrimental to many people, not just the patient. Patients, families, and healthcare professionals can all be affected by errors.

Effective systems must be in place to properly monitor for and detect nursing errors. These systems should be beneficial to all key stakeholders and add value to processes. Use of a just culture in an organization is also necessary for reporting, monitoring, and creating change.

Nurses should keep up to date with evidence-based practices. The use of bundles, developmental care considerations, and interdisciplinary rounding are all examples. As healthcare continues to evolve and research is done, changes in practice will continue to focus on what is learned to provide the best quality care to patients.

© The Author(s), under exclusive license to Springer Nature Switzerland AG 2025
K. Maryniak, *Controlling and Preventing Errors in Nursing Care of Pediatric Patients*, https://doi.org/10.1007/978-3-031-88185-5

MIX
Papier aus verantwortungsvollen Quellen
Paper from responsible sources
FSC® C105338

If you have any concerns about our products,
you can contact us on
ProductSafety@springernature.com

In case Publisher is established outside the EU,
the EU authorized representative is:
**Springer Nature Customer Service Center GmbH
Europaplatz 3, 69115 Heidelberg, Germany**

Printed by Libri Plureos GmbH
in Hamburg, Germany